3.12.79

New Age Training for Fitness and Health

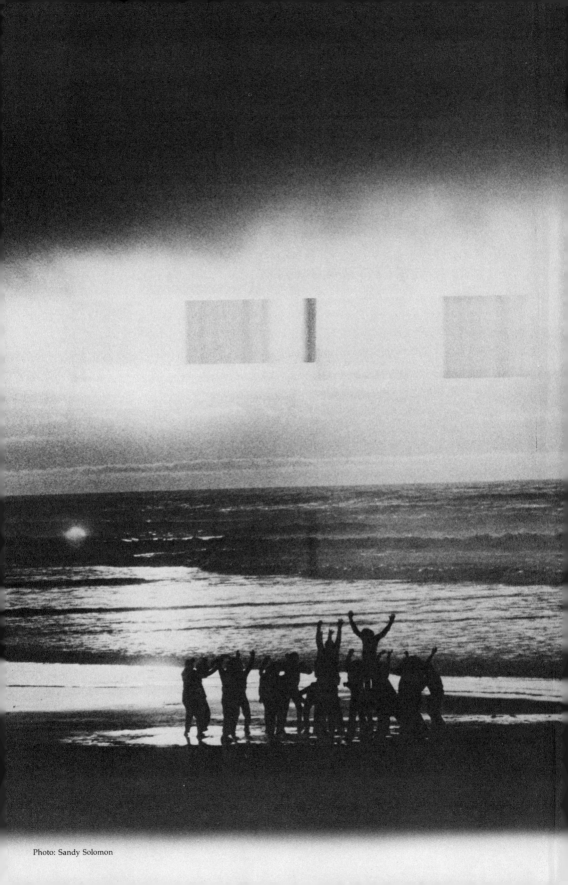

New Age Training for Fitness and Health

by Dyveke Spino

Grove Press, Inc.,
New York

First Edition 1979
First Printing 1979
ISBN: 0-394-50520-4
Grove Press ISBN: 0-8021-0177-1
Library of Congress Catalog Card Number: 78-65254

Library of Congress Cataloging in Publication Data

Spino, Dyveke
  New Age training for fitness and health.

  Includes index.
  1. Exercise. 2. Physical fitness. 3. Mind and body. 4. Physical education and training. I. Title.
RA781.S66   613.7'1   78-65254
ISBN 0-394-50520-4

Manufactured in the United States of America

Distributed by Random House, Inc., New York

GROVE PRESS, INC., 196 West Houston Street, New York, NY 10014

The author gratefully acknowledges permission to quote from the following:

Airola, Paavo. *Are You Confused?*, copyright 1971 by Paavo Airola, and *How To Get Well*. Health Plus Publishers, P.O. Box 22001, Phoenix, Arizona 85028.
Christensen, Alice and Rankin, David. *The Light of Yoga Society Beginner's Manual Yoga*, copyright © 1974 by Alice Christensen and David Rankin. Reprinted by permission of Simon & Schuster, a Division of Gulf and Western Corporation.
Gordon, Bill. "Blind Jogging," *Prevention Magazine*.
Kounovsky, Nicholas.
Laughingbird. "New Age Coach," *New Age Journal*, Feb. 1977.
Leonard, George. *The Ultimate Athlete*, copyright © 1974, 1975 by George Leonard. Reprinted by permission of Viking Penguin Inc.
Spino, Dyveke. "Creative Running," *New Age Journal*, Aug. 1977.
Sportelli, Louis, D. C. *Introduction to Chiropractic*, copyright © Louis Sportelli, D. C., 1978.

Book design: Edward Massengill.

Cover photo: Dyveke Spino and her daughter Terry Bryant.

This book is dedicated to my two children,
Terry and Stewart (Simon) Bryant,
and to Edward Massengill,
who have taught me the way of the Heart.

Contents

Acknowledgments

Any book is a writer's search for personal meaning. It is through Michael Murphy and George Leonard that I first became attuned to the theoretical basis of the mystical dimensions of sports which validated what I had experienced for many years. As we created the Esalen Sports Center, it was Percy Wells Cerutty's spirit that infused me with the heroic.

I wish to acknowledge the "special" people you will encounter in this book who have guided my work: Chuck Richardson, Jeanne Gibbs, Dr. Evarts Loomis, Dottie and Mel Morgan, Jim Waste, Jerry Mosher, and Vinita Bellandi.

My daughter, Terry, has been an invaluable spirit throughout, who always seemed to know the deepest of my intentions and helped me articulate them.

I feel very fortunate as a woman to have been married to a visionary City Planner/architect, Stewart G. Bryant, who not only became the father of my two beautiful children but who was a great teacher and inspiration. Stewart taught me the way of political responsibility and planetary ecology, with sensitivity and compassion.

To the healers and New Age therapists whose work helped me regain health and go on to coach others, I am indebted: Dr. William Baeza, Dr. Steve Bajon, Dr. Stephen Brown, Dr. Richard Kozlenko, Dr. Edward Jackson, Dr. Olga Worrell, Dr. Moshe Feldenkrais, and Othon Molina.

Others who provided support and inspiration were Peggy Taylor, Mark Bricklin, Richard Vogel, Gordon, and Leonard Ralston. And to my psychic and spiritual guides and teachers: Anne Armstrong, Helen Palmer, Walden Welch, and Dr. Robert Leichtman; I hope I have done justice in synthesizing the lessons they have taught me to help guide others.

I especially wish to acknowledge Dr. Stanley Krippner, Dr. John and Toni Lilly, and Robert and Nancy Monroe, whose pioneering work in human consciousness shattered my conceptions of human limitations. And I also deeply thank the hundreds of people in my private practice and workshops who permitted me to experiment with new and untried training methods.

My editor, Alan Rinzler, helped me to conceive the format and organization of the book and, along with the staff of Grove Press, directed it with love and professional competence.

I am deeply indebted to Creative Composition, Inc., Arlington, MA, the Atex Corporation, Bedford, MA, and Cosmos Press, New York City, for putting at my disposal the latest in computerized text processing and typesetting equipment. My use of this equipment provides a textbook example of the blending of the yin and the yang and greatly accelerated the writing of the book. My special thanks to Charles Ying of Atex, dreamer, visionary, and poet of the heart.

But it is Edward Massengill whom I honor and wish to acknowledge as the guiding force who provided me with the emotional support and intellectual brilliance which enabled me to share my life's work.

Dyveke Spino

New Age Training for Fitness and Health

Prelude to Living in the New Age

It is a cold December morning in Boston. Edward, a 40-year-old executive, is 15 minutes into a jog that is part of his Lifestyle Training Program. He is moving at about 12 miles per hour, just a little faster than a brisk walk. This keeps his pulse rate at around 150 beats per minute. Listen to his description of a transcendent run:

The Transcendent Run

I jog into a park where I usually run and make two circles around the large grassy area. The dew on the grass sparkles in the bright sunlight. I try to *experience* what is happening, not verbalize it.

I start my first run around the pond. The sun's reflection off the water is very bright; I can't even look at the pond in some places. I stop and run in place for a while and watch my friends, the ducks, as they drift away from me. I don't name them "ducks." I just see objects getting farther and farther away. I feel like running on the surface of the pond to follow them.

Now I start up into the woods. I run on leaves for a long time just experiencing the sound as my feet hit. I'm trying to concentrate on my feet today. I don't think "leaves," "feet." It is very important not to name. Once I name something and put it into a category, I turn off my sensory processes and miss the details.

I run up a path in the woods that leads to the crest of a hill overlooking the pond. Today I feel like doing an Indian dance. I imagine myself as an

Indian. Sounds of the type I associate with Indian dances come from deep in my abdomen. I *am* an Indian.

> *It is early in the morning and I am running through the woods. I get to the top of a hill. I want to invoke the blessings of the powers that affect my life and to give praise for the beauty around me. I see a tall tree with its top broken. The broken top is hanging by a thread at the side of the tree. I can imagine the force from the sky that struck the tree and I ask for protection from that power.*
>
> *I make a slow circle as I dance. I see many trees without leaves. I remember that this is a portent of cold and snow. I ask the spirits for warmth and food when that time comes. Now I see the lake through the trees; trees with green needles. The sun is shining down onto the lake. There are no words. I can only feel the beauty. I give praise to the powers that arranged this spectacle for me.*
>
> *Now I run around the crest of the hill for a while. I am slowly, relentlessly following the antelope which will furnish me with meat to satisfy my hunger and skin to protect me from the cold. I spot a valley that I haven't noticed before. I circle down into the valley and find a small body of water.*

As I run, I try to keep my mind clear to experience what is happening with my feet. I come out of the woods and go around the pond once in each direction. I begin the run from the park back to my house, all on asphalt pavement. I have plenty of breath but my legs don't want to move. I fasten my mind onto objects and stay focused on them as I run. First a streetlight. Then a Shell sign. And finally a red bell from Christmas decorations hung across the street. Each one of them is a target, a goal. My mind stays on the goal. Before I know it I'm at home taking a warm shower.

I have touched beauty today. I have touched one of my archetypal ancestors who lived hundreds of years ago. I lived in his shoes for a brief moment. I saw things in the uncluttered way he saw them. I really saw a tree, a squirrel, a lake, without imposing all my cultural restraints on them. I had a different conception of the cold, of how far a mile is, of how long an hour is. I lived in a different reality. I will never again take a tree for granted, a blade of grass, an oak leaf, a rock. As I ran, I participated in life. I left behind the trivia that usually fills my day and the overwhelming problems that sometimes leave me in despair. I have truly felt my connectedness to all of life.

Chapter One:
Living in the
New Age

One-Dimensional Living

Edward is an 40-year-old executive who, until about a year ago, was totally involved in his computer business. He had no time for aesthetics. He considered it a waste of time even to think about his environment. To him, a bedroom only needed a bed. Two white sheets and a blanket were fine. It didn't matter if the room had drapes, rugs, soft lighting: none of that contributed to the central function of the room, which was sleeping. He lived a Spartan existence consisting of little but work. He liked sports but never participated. He had always wanted to be an athlete but had long since given up on that. He hated the outdoors. "Why have the picnic at the park? Why not have it inside?" He would never walk if he could ride. He had to save all his energy for the business. He was living a focused life but there was no joy, beauty, excitement, or love.

He had started to run, but in a compulsive, masochistic way. It was always drudgery. He approached it the same way he approached his business: very seriously, no place for fun.

Edward attended one of my workshops because he wanted his fitness training to be fun. He got more than he had bargained for. His running not only became fun, in the sense that he now enjoys doing it, but he also began to identify with nature and the beauty of the outdoors. He started to transcend his everyday existence and get in touch with another reality. His focus was no longer solely on physical training, but on developing his faculties to the fullest degree. He began to apply the feminine principle to all aspects of his life. In short, he started a Lifestyle Training Program.

Most people are like Edward. They lead one-dimensional lives. They don't partake fully of what life has to offer. Those who begin a physical training program often do it in the same one-dimensional way they live the rest of their lives, and in most cases drop out of training after a short while. The key idea of New Age coaching is to use physical training to continually ignite a joyous and transcendent life. Without that, we might as well be training robots. Part of my job is to help ignite you in the midst of the crushing reality of life that is smothering your higher faculties. You cannot expect these transcendent experiences to occur predictably or regularly without systematic training. And you cannot expect to reach these experiences in a body that is polluted, toxic, overweight, misaligned, and out of shape.

Evoking Transcendent Experiences

I am a coach, but not the kind of coach you may remember from high school. I call myself a New Age Coach. I was one of the founders of the Esalen Sports Center and have studied and done pioneering training work with the forerunners in the mystical approach to sports, including Michael Murphy, founder of Esalen, George Leonard, and Percy Wells Cerutty, master Australian Olympic coach.

Currently, I travel all over the country working with various professional and business organizations. My approach is to blend methods and techniques from the Eastern and mystical traditions with modern sports training methods to heighten athletic excellence, lifestyle awareness, and inner exploration. I design specific individualized programs to help people become *athletes in training*.

In beginning my work as a New Age coach, I had no role models to follow, no curriculum or precedent. Through an evolutionary process that started with my own confusion and personal struggle to find health and vitality, I was sent on a search for another way. This search led me away from competitive sports that damaged my body and induced a sense of separation from others, away from those medical practitioners who seemed bent on carving me up and prescribing drugs.

My path led me, albeit circuitously, to desire to inspire people to reach for the upper limits of human functioning, to be in touch with their feelings, in touch with the wonder of life, and to nurture and tend this process with love and compassion. I wanted to help others penetrate and expand their consciousness through discipline, awareness, and, above all else, a oneness with nature.

I myself needed a physical training program that did not view the body as a competitive machine; a program in which athletic disciplines could balance the masculine and feminine aspects of my being; in which inner power could be released through mystical and artistic endeavors, and in which I could experience personal *transcendence*.

I knew that I had touched magical moments of inner beauty and outer harmony on the tennis court and the ski slope, diving off a diving board, swimming a pounding ocean surf. These moments and my daily runs on Mt. Tamalpais were precious. I felt that I had touched some ancient wisdom deep within my cellular system that had somehow become inarticulate in our culture; a wisdom that regarded the athlete as a sacred vessel offering his or her physical skill as a form of divine worship.

My early training as a concert pianist, under the tutelege of my aunt at the Peabody Conservatory of Music, was interwoven with a passionate desire for sports and games. My mother, an opera singer and dancer with Isadora Duncan, went to live in Java with her husband, a Danish surgeon, who established a hospital to work with lepers. At the age of five, I went to live with my aunt to pursue music and academic studies at the conservatory.

There seemed a natural linkage between the study and discipline of music, in which there is a sense of flow, beauty, and interweaving, and the rhythms and tempos that I experienced as a physically active young woman. The brilliance of Mozart, the compression and condensation of Bartok, the pathos of Chopin, the lilting grace of Scarlatti, the majestic elevation of Bach, were similar to what I experienced when moving my body in sports. Emotions were triggered, surges of power would pour into my psyche, and I would experience complete joy; a sense of transcending all the boundaries and beliefs of temporal limitations. At times I felt flooded by spiritual energy from a source I did not understand, giving me a finer sensitivity to the qualities of human aspirations.

As a New Age Coach, part of my job is to help people learn how to structure their environments to afford the most opportunities for these transcendent experiences. It is possible for us to achieve our highest aspirations. We can transcend our mundane world through beauty and love. Becoming a New Age person essentially means learning to restructure our reality so that it contains these transcendent experiences. This is what I call the *feminine principle*.

Thus, a training program to prepare a person to live in the New Age is not a *physical* training program alone. Rather, it is a *Total Lifestyle* Training Program. It must involve the whole person: getting the body aligned, moving the body, cleaning up nutrition, learning to visualize, training the will. Great strength and total awareness are necessary for living in the New Age. Only a training program that deals with your total lifestyle can prepare you for that life.

The goal of a Lifestyle Training Program is not only to show you that the you can touch moments of transcendence, but also that those moments can be *purposely evoked*.

New Age Coach

My job as a New Age Coach is also to train people to live in the New Age. A New Age person is one who has achieved a balance between the male and female energies present in all of us; one who can evoke joy, beauty, love, in himself or herself and in those around them. A New Age person identifies with every form of life in both the vegetable and animal kingdoms and feels an interconnectedness with all living things. A New Age person tries to achieve the fullest expression of himself or herself.

Reaching this ideal will require the systematic training of the body, mind, and spirit. It requires dealing with what Maslow calls the *higher needs*: ultimate values, peak experiences, transcendence (rising above) of the self, oneness, maximal sensory awareness, maximal interpersonal encounter, cosmic awareness, ecstasy, awe. Physical training and physical fitness are only one aspect of New Age coaching. They are actually only a means to the greater end of fully expressing ourselves at all levels.

In Chapter Five, *Awakening the Feminine Principle*, I will outline the processes of developing these faculties in the context of physical exercise. These abilities to evoke transcendent experiences emerge from the *will to evoke ecstasy*, to balance the culture we are living in. A culture that is weary of war, drugs, overstimulation. We are desperately looking for *simple, exquisite ways that are personal and self-directed to obtain magical moments and help us integrate and reaffirm the beauty of life.*

Though I work with many groups at conferences, workshops, and seminars, some of my most satisfying experiences have resulted from my work with individuals. Among my students have been notables such as George Leonard, who features my work in his book *The Ultimate Athlete*, Mark Bricklin, Editor of *Prevention* magazine, Donald Ardel and Dr. John Travis of *High Level Wellness*, Peggy Taylor, Editor of *New Age Journal*. Bill Turque of NBC News filmed a documentary of my work on Mount Tamalpais and ended up on a training program I devised for him.

I have coached parapsychologist Dr. Stanley Krippner; psychics Dr. Helen Palmer and Anne Armstrong; psychiatrist Dr. Jerry Jampolsky; and the *father of holistic medicine*, Dr. Evarts Loomis, surgeon and homeopathic doctor. I have conducted training sessions for Stanley Keleman, Robert Monroe, Dr. John Lilly, Dr. Leonard Duhl, Dr. Norman Shealey, and Gay Luce. I set up a running and tennis program for Daniel and Pat Ellsberg. My most intense coaching relationship was with Jim Waste, long-distance runner and coach to the Bay Area Touring Side Rugby Team, which is equivalent to a US Olympic team.

But most of my clients are men and women who are neither famous nor athletes. Each has come from a different vantage point: to start a program, overcome injury-producing habits, clear up psychological blocks, "get their lives together." I have worked with corporation lawyers, secretaries, university professors, nurses, and many doctors and psychiatrists. Some of my clients are high school students, injured psychologically by authoritarian coaches or difficult home situations. Others have been physically handicapped or have had learning disabilities or shattered emotions. I usually end up *coaching* anyone with whom I'm affiliated personally or professionally.

I want you to share this path. I want to help you devise your own Lifestyle Training Program based on your own needs. On the one hand we all need a personal coach — someone to help guide us through a learning process. But since I can't be with each of you in person, I want to use this book to help you become an *Athlete in Training*, which includes becoming a creative artist of the soul.

In an attempt to disseminate the inspiration and information that can lead to optimal health, I founded an institute, *New Dimensions in Lifestyle*. The purpose of this institute is to help more people reach optimal health, fitness, and awareness. I am especially interested in using my skills with corporations. There could be vast increases in motivation and job performance and a considerable saving of human lives by incorporating enlightened health and fitness programs based on lifestyle reeducation into a company's structure.

One by-product of coaching people to live in the New Age is the hastening of the coming of the New Age. When executives learn to evoke the feminine principle in their lives, they will no longer be able to justify having the employees work in sterile environments with fluorescent lights and no place to recharge their energy.

The Brain and the Feminine Principle

To understand the feminine principle, it is helpful to have some of the latest information as to how the brain functions.

Our brains have two hemispheres: a left hemisphere and a right hemisphere. The left, or masculine hemisphere, contains the speech center. It is through this side of the brain that we think in concepts, that we use linear deductive reasoning processes. This logical, deductive aspect is the basis of our educational system. The left hemisphere of the brain is intellectual, reductionistic, and the center for analysis and rational thinking. Most of us are masculine in orientation. Our functioning is geared toward execution of action to realize specific goals in a logical and analytical fashion.

Most of the books on physical training are written by men and have a left-hemisphere orientation: train the body as an efficient machine to compete better, either with oneself or others. The underlying value is competition.

Physically training the body as a machine, following log books and specific schedules, can help you to develop a finely tuned system. But there is more to the human experience than mechanistic efficiency. We also live in a world of feelings.

The right hemisphere of the brain is the hemisphere of the *feminine principle*, the location of the language of feelings. Its characteristics are quite different from the intellectual, reductionistic, analytic mode of functioning of the left hemisphere. The right side of the brain is sensuous, intuitive, *feels* in a comprehensive way the totality of a situation, synthesizes information instantly without deductive reasoning, and awakens you to the fullest aspects of your being. Many inventors, scientists, mathematicians, artists, and musicians have their most important breakthroughs from the right hemisphere when knowledge is revealed in dreams, intuitions, sudden flashes.

The right hemisphere dictates the laws of relatedness, of human emotions, and governs the inner or spiritual world. Thus, the feminine principle cannot be understood through an intellectual or academic approach. The real meaning of things evades any direct interrogation. Information is often revealed in mysterious ways, through symbolic, intuitive, and sometimes seemingly illogical processes. The feminine principle is concerned with *fertility*, human growth, inner awareness, spiritual aspiration, and with an instinctively protective and nurturing attitude toward all life, a sense of the connectedness and oneness of all living things.

Awakening the feminine principle opens the psychic abilities of the right hemisphere of the brain. In my case, my *sensing* abilities are a way of instantaneously getting information from other than logical or deductive reasoning. My clairvoyant gifts allow me to see and relate to the person who is in the process of transformation. I relate to him as though that transition has already happened.

I have systematically trained these abilities. In my coaching I use altered states of consciousness to gain information about clients, to organize events. Sometimes I get flashes about events that later materialize. I believe there is a direct relationship between developing one's athletic and artistic gifts and heightening the special powers of the mind. In consultations I sometimes have an overwhelming sense of understanding the complexity of another's life. In coaching sessions, I sometimes feel in my body areas of pain or trauma in the other person.

It is always difficult to describe these nebulous psychic impressions, just as it is difficult to describe feelings aroused by a piece of music. It is a feeling state of instantaneous knowingness without inhibition or self-consciousness. I've learned to trust the spontaneity of the moment and rely on my psychic and intuitive gifts as an artist of the moment. I never have a set plan or rote speech, whether I'm speaking before one or a thousand. I allow the free play of the group's energy to call forth the appropriate mode of sharing my knowledge. I take everything into consideration: mood, tone, feeling, environment, attraction and repulsion between people. I always extend boundaries. Extending physical boundaries extends personal boundaries.

I am not only a New Age coach: I am a woman. I speak from an androgynous perspective; a perspective that includes both the masculine and the feminine principles of human functioning. This book is different from all the other books on physical training and exercise in that it is concerned with helping you to construct an individually tailored lifestyle training program. None of the other books deal with awakening the *feminine principle* while disciplining the body in a physical endeavor.

This is not to imply that the others are invalid or insignificant. Cooper's books on aerobic conditioning turned the country on to the importance of cardiovascular training. Leonard's and Pritikin's *Live Longer Now* outlines a simple formula of exercise and diet. They show how longevity can be increased by controlling the degenerative diseases through lifestyle changes. There is a vast array of fine books about specific training, sequential programs, and testing devices to measure your level of physical performance. But none of these books refers to the simultaneous physical training of the body and the awakening of the inner state of being.

I want to speak to you as a New Age coach and a woman; to awaken you to the *feminine principle*, and to help you design your own Lifestyle Training Program from the perspective of blending the masculine and feminine sides of your personality. Such an approach is personified in the *Vitalistic Theory of Health* which is based on *synthesis of the whole person*.

The Place of the Feminine Principle

Our attitudes towards physical exercise and sports have come from the military tradition of ancient cultures which developed our bodies for war against another tribe or nation, to win territorial boundaries, to compete with an enemy or gain control of resources and thus have the power to dominate. Competition has infused most of the books about physical exercise and sports training. Little or minimal attention has been paid to the higher aspirations of the human spirit.

We simply cannot continue our predominantly masculine view of the universe. We cannot treat ourselves or our natural resources as endlessly expendable any more than we can drop nuclear bombs on other countries or dump nuclear wastes in our oceans. This is the archaic *hunter instinct of the warrior* from which our attitudes toward physical training and sports have come.

I believe it is time for women to step forward and become true leaders of the New Age, visionaries who blend the *feminine principle* into all our insitutional structures. It is time for women to draw forth from the consciousness of men the capacity to be in touch with the oneness of life, to be in touch with their feelings, with the highest of human aspirations: protecting and nurturing their bodies and their planet as one living organism.

And I believe that it is time for women to systematically discipline and train their bodies as beautiful instruments of the New Age, to learn to assert themselves with love and wisdom and guide the major decision-making processes of our culture. This means learning to handle stress, becoming a courageous, balanced, harmonious woman, who believes in her power and has the physical endurance and flexibility to withstand the incredible stresses these changes imply.

Vitalistic Health

A vitalistic theory of health views the universe as an interchangeable system of energy, and the human body as connected to everything else: rocks, the sea, each other. It is based upon the idea of *interconnectedness*, "relatedness," and thus centers upon the feminine principle. A vitalistic approach to health, to exercise, and lifestyle fitness includes the feminine principle which can help you evolve toward your fullest humanity.

A vitalistic theory sees life as a mystery and the quality of life as being of an artistic nature. Health grows, therefore, out of a state of being. Health is derived from integrity of the system. Feelings and sensations must be awakened. Intuitive self-reflection must become a part of your daily life. Poetry, music, sculpture, sunsets, beauty must awaken your spirit to your highest aspirations. You must learn to weep with tenderness and know Dionysian explosions of joy.

This is what a *vitalistic* view of health must reflect. This is what I hope to inspire you to build into a daily Lifestyle Training Program; awakening the right hemisphere of your brain while simultaneously training your physical body. What makes this book different from others is the synthesis and application of these ideas, methods, and training principles, which I have used in the lives of hundreds of others.

Stress

Life is a strange paradox. On one hand, each of us values ourself, knows our worth and demands attention in the eyes and opinions of others. Yet, there is a *dark side*, the self-destructive side, that sometimes arises with power quite beyond our conscious control. We do things that we know can cause catastrophic damage to our bodies. We surround ourselves with energies that deplete and drain us. But we know full well that there is something greater, more beautiful inside us waiting to be touched, unveiled, listened to, ignited by a compassionate moment of true understanding; perhaps love.

Of course, I couldn't write these words if I didn't know the same paradox in my own life. How could I presume to have anything to offer you unless I had been subject to all the same lessons? I am fragile. I am vulnerable. I am heroic though at times frightened. And there's a quiet voice inside me saying, "Pay attention to yourself, have courage to believe in yourself, and reach toward your inner beauty, connect your inner awakening to your physical health so that you can better handle the stress in your life." If you want to listen to that voice, this book can help you.

Much of the stress in our lives is based on the masculine principle of human functioning which has dominated the world for thousands of years. And it is most highly manifested in the competition present in our sports and games. Competition in the finest sense should imply reaching for the upper limits of perfection, self-mastery, real inner wisdom. In many cases it does. And certainly not all competition is bad. But, as it is generally applied in our culture, it is extremely destructive and we know the results all too well.

How many business executives do you know who drink themselves to bad health in the evenings and on weekends? How many women learn to battle for survival in their professional advancement and lose a certain softness? How many children are left untouched and unloved because of parents too busy *getting up the ladder*? And how many psyches of young people are damaged in their academic years through athletic endeavors because they *couldn't make it*? Or worse, how many are injured for life? For example, there are 50,000 knee operations a year on high school children who play football.

A New View of Health

We live in a society that equates *not being sick enough to go to a doctor* with being *healthy*. We go to a doctor when there is a symptom so serious that we can't handle it ourselves. The doctor treats that symptom and usually helps us get rid of it. We don't see him again until there is another such symptom or until we have a periodic medical checkup. At the checkup, the doctor takes our pulse, our blood pressure, weighs us and puts us through a series of tests. But unfortunately, his *OK* doesn't signify that we are in optimal health.

For example, what about the headache that seems to be triggered whenever some stressful situation occurs? Two or three aspirin may take care of it temporarily, but it keeps coming back. Even though it's not bad enough to call a doctor, there's no doubt that such an occurrence is not consistent with optimal health. What about that pain in the side? He says, "Don't worry. It's just a muscle spasm." But he doesn't say what to do about it, and it keeps coming back. What about the tenseness in the body when something is going wrong at work? The body gets as tight as a wound-up spring. A tinge of fear is present. An irritability surfaces.

What about the pain in the back that appears every few months and makes life miserable for a week or so and then disappears? What about the cigarette smoke going into the lungs every day, shortening the life span? What about the excess alcohol being consumed? What about the feeling of uselessness that occurs when retirement is contemplated? The list of things going wrong for so-called *healthy* people is interminable. And this is only the tip of the iceberg.

What if you could look 45 when you're actually 60? What if you could *feel* 40 when you're actually 50? Wouldn't it be great to be able to play tennis, swim, run, dance, hike without becoming totally exhausted and without a continual series of injuries? Wouldn't it be exciting to have so much energy that you couldn't wait to play basketball with your kids? Wouldn't you be happy if you could once more approach your job with enthusiasm? Imagine having so much energy that sex is no longer an effort after a day of work and an evening of fun? Imagine having enough energy to extend the care you have for yourself and your immediate family to others outside your family. Picture yourself at 70, not creeping around with a cane, bound by stiff muscles and brittle bones, but running the 26-plus miles of a marathon as if you were a 30-year-old.

These considerations suggest what optimal health means. But to whom do we turn for information about how to live with optimal health? Those who consult their local doctor about getting into better health usually find that it is pretty impossible to get information, not to mention inspiration. The doctor can help you get rid of a tumor, an appendix, or control your diabetes with insulin, but is just too busy to spend much time with you if you aren't obviously ill. And even if doctors had the time, they probably don't have anything like all the information necessary to help the patient alter lifestyle patterns so as to reach optimal health.

We have made the mistake of approaching health from the wrong direction. We have accepted the view that there are experts *out there* who can help us have good health. So we turn health matters over to them. It is true that there are specialists who can help us with specific problems. There is the cardiologist for heart problems, the podiatrist for foot problems, the chiropractor for spinal alignment problems, the psychiatrist or psychologist for emotional problems, the optometrist or ophthalmologist for eye problems. There is seemingly no end of such experts. And now there are new therapies such as rolfing, a technique to get the body properly aligned with gravity. There are ancient therapies such as acupuncture and yoga that are finally being accepted as new health options.

But we expect too much of the specialists. Just because a doctor can help us with a foot problem doesn't mean he is qualified to help us reach optimal health. Any individual practitioner seems to have only part of the answer. Life and health are certainly better in many ways because of these experts, but we take the wrong approach when we expect these specialists to help us with the more general problem.

Individuals must begin to take responsibility for their own health. They must have enough concern about their most valuable asset, health, to start and maintain a workable program. They need to (1) learn about the options available, (2) identify the aspects of their personal health that need attention, (3) begin immediately to lay the base for health, and (4) build a support network that will sustain this quest for optimal health. It is too much to expect an individual to be able to put together his or her own program alone. Fortunately, there is an emerging body of work which can help.

Ironically, perhaps, this approach to optimal health comes not from the medical community concerned with specialization and pathology, but from individuals in other disciplines such as nutrition, biochemistry, physics, and especially from scientists involved in research in endurance training. This is especially true in the field of running. Those who pursue running in a serious way tend to become addicted and want to tune up the body for better performance. They start to think about nutrition, about how to avoid injuries and pain. Many start to have emotional releases during running as they begin to tune in to the majesty of nature. Some begin to give serious consideration to their environment and lifestyle. This represents a movement toward a holistic approach to health.

A typical corporation spends hundreds of dollars a year per employee for medical insurance premiums. Some corporations are now beginning to be concerned not only about protecting an employee's finances from ever-rising medical expenses, but also about helping the employees alter the conditions that lead to hospitalization. They are beginning to be interested in helping employees upgrade their physical condition, deal with on-the-job stress, prepare for retirement.

The Health Coach

This approach by corporations is in total harmony with a newly emerging concept of health: that health is not merely the *absence* of disease but is, in addition, the *presence* of adequate endurance, flexibility, strength, and mental powers to fully participate in and enjoy life. This approach has led to a new profession, the *Health Coach*. The Health Coach helps individuals take responsibility for their health and instructs them in laying the necessary physical and mental base.

The Health Coach is quite different from the traditional coach we're so familiar with: the coach who diligently studies films of last week's game, puts his athletes through agonizing workouts, has them shot up with drugs to coax out one more performance, shuffles human beings as if they were plastic chess pieces. The Health Coach is concerned with helping individuals discover their motivational ignition switch and alter their lifestyle to reach *optimal health, fitness and awareness*.

Whereas traditional coaches are concerned with the most promising athletes: the person who can throw a baseball 95 miles per hour, kick a football 80 yards, or run a mile in 3:50, the Health Coach is open to anyone. The Health Coach is interested in the unhappy 12-year-old child who is 15 pounds overweight and whose father is *too busy* to talk to him. The Health Coach is concerned with the woman who feels bad about her body, who sits at a desk all day drinking diet colas and trying every new diet fad in a effort to stay slim. The Health Coach is concerned with the 40-year-old executive who is committing slow suicide with too many cigarettes, too much red meat, alcohol, and stress. The Health Coach is concerned with the 50-year-old who is feeling a definite decline in physical fitness and is starting the slow but sure slide to retirement, obsolescence, and a feeling of uselessness.

The Health Coach realizes that it is up to individuals to take responsibility for their health but also realizes that individuals need help in getting started. The Health Coach has a health overview to impart to individuals who want to take charge and begin to lay the base for optimal health. The Health Coach knows that optimal health must be viewed in terms of a person's entire lifestyle. The Health Coach must introduce the person systematically to the natural processes of living that will not only prevent disease, aging, breakdown through stress and negative addictive patterns, but will lead to positive daily living that can result in optimal health.

One of my special functions as a New Age Coach is serving as a Health Coach for my clients.

How You Can Change Your Life

Just as in nature the *Great Spirit* has cycles, so do you. To prepare for these cycles of change that press upon us, we need tools to develop our inner power through endurance, flexibility, and a sense of self-transcendence. I want to share my methods and *spirit* and help you to devise your own program and keep it flexible enough to reflect the ebbs and flows of your life. You see, the feminine principle includes the changeability of human nature. I hope to assist you in assessing your lifestyle with clarity and precision that will help you determine how you can fit a training program into your schedule.

In Chapter 2, you will have the opportunity to assess your total lifestyle: how you spend your time, what your nutrition is like, what kind of home and work environments you have, who you would like to be if you could have your wildest dream.

It is also imperative to *train your will*, the intentionality of your life-force, and use it wisely and skillfully in propelling you effortlessly toward your goals. I discuss this in Chapter 3 which is based on the ideas of Roberto Assagioli. I have used these ideas extensively in helping others start and maintain a Lifestyle Training Program and have designed simple tools based on these principles for use in your training program.

As a coach, I hope to awaken your natural physical spirit through five areas of conditioning of mind, body, and spirit. The five areas, explored in a holistic fashion are: endurance, strength, flexibility, sensing, and innerspace. Chapter 4 will discuss moving the body and Chapter 5 will deal with sensing and innerspace. Chapter 6 will help you start a proper nutrition program. Chapter 7 will show you how to bring your body into proper alignment and keep it flexible.

There are biological and psychological differences between men and women which affect both implementation and maintenance of a training program. In Chapters 8 and 9, I will explore these conceptually and through case studies and weave my insights with materials from psychology, music, intuition, and experience. In Chapter 10, I will discuss New Age Graduate Training, broadening the parameters of a Lifestyle Training Program. And in Chapter 11, I will summarize how to design your own personal Lifestyle Training Program and talk about my visions of tomorrow and the Coach of the Future.

A Lifestyle Training Program must first and foremost begin with *accepting yourself*. As Percy Cerutty said to me many times, "Believe in yourself, trust yourself, and never, never quit."

You have a unique world view, a unique reality, that results from the way you are building your life. You have unique problems and sometimes you feel overwhelmed and discouraged. This is not a program to pit you against yourself, but to help you to love yourself.

You are delicate and fragile at times, needing compassion and care. There may be a time when you push to your upper limits and go over the edge and pull a hamstring, sprain an ankle, break a limb. You may feel frightened that you are overweight and maybe shouldn't begin a training program, or fearful that you may start a program, discontinue it, and then feel bad about yourself. You may be a harried middle-aged executive, saturated with hotels, stress, family problems, and restaurant food.

But I have touched many dark and secret places in the lives of people I have coached. I have seen heroic moments of impossible excellence. All of that is there for you to touch, marvel at, and respect. Fitness is not something you *do*, not a regimen of *standards of perfection* plucked arbitrarily from a book. Fitness is a way of life, part of a total lifestyle. It is a way for everything that you do to go better. I extend my hand to you. I want to take your hand and help you begin this joyous journey.

I hope to inspire you to start a Lifestyle Training Program. It is not 30 minutes a week, or three times a week, fast and quick. Health, vitality, inspiration, a sense of dedication to *loving yourself* is a Lifestyle commitment. You are developing your body as a temple of the spirit and this includes not only enhancing your physical body, but also enhancing your finer qualities of character and aiming your life's path toward personal ecology and planetary responsibility.

This book is being written, in part, to counterbalance the overabundance of books on physical conditioning and sports that are written only from one perspective: training the physical body to be an *efficient machine* that can compete better, either with yourself or others.

The *feminine principle* has one essential precept: each of us is a part of a system which is interconnected to everything in the universe. The *feminine principle* deals with the *inner person*. To deal only with the *outer body* from a totally masculine or linear left-brain perspective, as most sport and physical training books do, is to divert us from using our training time to unlock the recesses of wonder within us.

The Loving Human Being

As a New Age Coach, I want to help you develop into a loving human being who will nurture and support your life processes so as to approach your fullest humanness. This necessitates viewing your body not as a competitive machine but as a vehicle to integrate the masculine and feminine aspects of your being and to enable you to experience your own personal transcendence.

As Rolling Thunder, American Indian healer and spiritual teacher, expresses it:

> It's very important for people to realize that the earth is a living organism, the body of a higher individual who has a will and wants to be well, who is at times less healthy or more healthy, physically and mentally. People should treat their own bodies with respect. It's the same thing with the earth. Too many people don't know that when they harm the earth they harm themselves. Nor do they realize that when they harm themselves they harm the earth. Some of the people interested in ecology want to protect the earth and yet they will cram anything into their mouths just for tripping or for freaking out — even using some of our sacred agents. Some of these things I call helpers and they are very good if they are taken very, very seriously. But they have to be used in the right way or they'll be useless and harmful. And most people don't know about these things. All these things have to be understood.

> It's not very easy for you people to understand these things because understanding is not knowing the kind of facts that your books and teachers talk about. I can tell you that understanding begins with love and respect. It begins with respect for the Great Spirit. And the Great Spirit is the life that is in all things; all the creatures and the plants and even the rocks and the minerals. All things, and I mean *all* things, have their own will and their own way and their own purpose. This is what is to be respected.

Such respect is not a feeling or an attitude only. It's a way of life. Such respect means that we never stop realizing and never neglect to carry out our obligation to ourselves and our environment.

Prelude to Asking "Who Am I?"

Many of us live a lifestyle with set habits and ritualistic ways of relating to our external environment. We don't particularly pay attention to whether there are fluorescent lights in the place we work, whether we drive through congested traffic and noise that sap our energy, or whether we constantly eat in a hurry and with little attention to what we are putting in our digestive system. We are creatures of habit and before we can begin a lifestyle geared to health, fitness, and awareness, we must sit back and reflect on the options available to alter these patterns in ways that can bring about an entirely new pattern of well-being.

Mark's Consultation

Mark, 44, a typical Type A executive driven by high stress during the day, too many demands on his time, a jammed brief case on the weekends, martinis and bourbons between lunch and dinner to relieve headaches and low back pain, is a good example of the type of man who comes to my home in Mill Valley, California, for an evening consultation.

For these consultations, I arrange the environment to be soothing and relaxing, sometimes with soft music, candles, the lights turned low, and a fire going. Across the room I watched this rather bent and out-of-alignment body take off an overcoat and hat and sit down in the rocking chair, utterly fatigued. The first day the furrow in his forehead stayed for a full 30 minutes before I could see his muscles finally relax and let go. He evidently went through every day as though primed for attack.

When clients first come to me to be coached, it is necessary for me to keep the tone of the interchange intimate and free of distractions. I always create an aesthetic environment to awaken their sense of personal inspiration and inner power. I want to help them reflect on their current lifestyles and to allow a free-flowing stream of consciousness. Not only does this environment allow me to tune into their nuances and the subleties of their lives, but I can become connected with them at a personal level and watch the various roles and external expectations drop away.

I sat back as I said to Mark, "I don't know anything about you, but paint me a picture in 45 minutes to an hour. Tell me who you are, what's important to you, what's going on in your life, something about your fears, your dreams, your quiet aspirations. Paint me a picture as though I'm a stranger and I need to get an overall picture of who you are, a biographical sketch." I just sat back, flipped on the tape recorder, and, almost before I could finish asking the question, I watched Mark take a deep breath, unclench his fists, stretch out his legs, and organize his internal system of functioning to allow his own personal self-report system to flow.

Mark started:

> All I ever wanted to be when I was a young boy and in college was a great success in the business world. I wanted to earn over $50,000 a year and have many employees under me. I wanted to dominate and control and I learned to be very good at it. I was driving and hard-working. Some people even called me a workaholic. I had a natural flair that created an independent streak in me and I didn't want to work for somebody else if I could be my own boss. So I found I was always doing the extra thing to get ahead, to push a little bit harder. I'd take extra reports home, travel a bit further for business meetings and conferences.
>
> My wife was good at details, at running the house, taking care of the kids. I guess it's the old pattern. I was out being the business success. She was home taking care of all the details and feeling very unfulfilled as a woman.
>
> I found more and more that I started to drink socially to close business deals, to make contacts, and to get away from the stress of the day. And I began to find during the last three or four years that the noon martini started to get into an afternoon syndrome that often went through the evening and far more than I would like to admit to. And it is getting so that now if I don't have alcohol in the house all the time, I feel something is missing.
>
> In some ways I've gotten to the top. I'm 44. I make from 30 to 50 thousand a year. I have four children, a nice house, car, pleasant enough life, but I'm truly not happy inside. And the awful thing is that I'm beginning to have to take more and more aspirin every day to get through the hangover of the morning. And I'm smoking too many cigarettes. I'm faced with a real crisis now because I have very little in common with my wife, very little contact with the children — they're growing now — and I really want to get into more meaningful work, something more humanitarian, that has to do with people rather than making money.

I thought of all the Marks who had come through my living room with basically the same story, each a variation on a theme.

I asked Mark if he had any physical problems. He told me about a knee problem and a lower back problem. He had gradually stopped playing tennis and skiing because of these physical difficulties and didn't think anything could be done about it.

> I started to gain weight. At first it was only five or ten pounds and then it slipped up to 15, 18, and now that I'm about 30 pounds overweight, I find it very hard to do the athletic things I used to do. I tried to play baseball with the kids the other day and run around the bases. I was so out of breath I could barely make home plate. I was really ashamed. I thought, "What a price I've paid to be so successful. My body is falling apart. I don't relate to my children. I hardly have sex with my wife anymore. I'm not internally happy."

His voice trailed off. He wasn't seeking overt sympathy. I was very impressed with the candid truthfulness that came out almost instantaneously. I have found this repeatedly to be the case. Once people are willing to do a self-assessment of their lifestyle, they didn't want to pussy-foot around or paint the kind of fictitious picture they have to the rest of the day. They want to tell it as it is, truthfully, bluntly.

> I was very active physically as a young student, played on basketball and tennis teams through college, was in excellent physical condition, married shortly out of college and went to work for a big corporation. I Worked very hard for the first ten to 15 years, to the exclusion of very much family time, and fell into a pattern of the occasional love affairs that would pull me away from too much intimacy with the family, with my wife. That was secondary. The most important thing was that I had "gotten out of touch with my feelings."

> I know I'm a sugar-holic. I'm addicted to coffee and aspirins and I know I eat too much junk food. But I don't know what else to do. It's just a habit and it's easy. In the last three years I've had a lot of trouble with my right knee and lower back and some problems with indigestion and constipation. Not bad enough that I've needed serious medication, but I just know that everything's out of whack. I don't feel high or good much of the time and frankly I'm concerned about my wife's health as well as my own because she doesn't get any exercise at all and seems to be getting a little bitchier every year.

> I feel like I'm on a treadmill and I know that my health is really going to give out on me.

I asked Mark how he would like to live his life if he could have his wildest dream. And then I sat back and watched his eyes sparkle, his hands gesture, and the rocking chair start to sway.

> Oh God, in my wildest dream I'd chuck the whole thing. I'd give up the house, I'd give up all those cars, the boat, and I'd really get my body and my mind together. I'd get closer to the earth and the natural things of life that I feel so cut off from.

If I had my wildest dream, I think it would have something to do with the sea. I've always wanted to study oceanography and I used to do skin diving. I think it would be wonderful to get a boat and for us all to learn to live a much more natural life. I want to get down to the real thing, studying how the sea works, how the life of the sea works, and to get my family back to the natural elements. I want to get the pollution out of my lungs and out of my body and cells and get my mind in a better space. I want to earn a living, keep my family together and still do socially useful work. Well that's what my wildest dream is.

Mark had shared an amazing amount of information in an hour and 20 minutes. He sat forward and said, "Dyveke, I have a feeling that tonight is a beginning. I have a feeling there is real hope for me, that I just don't have to go down the drain like so many of my other friends and die of a heart attack at 55 or 57, that I don't have to watch my family fall apart. I really want to get my body and my mind together and be do things in this world that turn me on and make me happy every day."

We stood up. I walked him to the door, took his hand and said, "You know, Mark, you replace every cell in your body in three years and every cell in your central nervous system every seven years. Do you realize that in three years, with proper training and nutrition, you can be a totally different human being?" He smiled and went outside. As the moon cast its light on him he said, "I'm really ready to try."

Chapter Two:
Asking "Who Am I?"

Getting Ready for Your Lifestyle Review

Your training program is a very personal and unique work of art, which will be sculptured and reshaped by trial and error. You will need to accept the feminine principle which is based upon *changeability*. Although you will chart a course with specific times and activities, you need to understand that the schedule cannot always be met. You will be steering your life as though on uncharted seas and sometimes you will be "blown astray" by trips, friends, unexpected meetings, injuries. It is essential to be accepting and self-appreciative during these times.

I cannot stress how important it is to accept from the start that at times your training schedule will need *alternatives*. As a coach, I find the creativity involved in altering the training course is just as important as creating it. Flexibility in scheduling takes self-knowledge based on personal assessment through a continuous process of evaluation and reflection. Your training program will include such a process of continuous self-examination.

In this section I will share with you some of the important variables to consider in assessing your life. This assessment process is part of my many years of coaching people individually. The insights I have gained have guided me in condensing the areas around which you will need to focus.

Building the Foundation

The Lifestyle Assessment you will experience in this chapter is the foundation upon which your training program will be built. It includes an assessment of your schedule, your environment, and friendship network. You will examine how you spend evenings and weekends, what training resources are available, what equipment for your home or office could facilitate your program. You will analyze how you are "filling your mind" and what is energizing and depleting you.

You will complete a nutritional profile that will help you clean up your eating habits by making you aware of what you're eating and why. I am also including a brief synopsis and profile on healing arts that will introduce you to natural ways of dealing with total vitalistic health, and ways of overcoming injuries or illness; in short, *to promote high level wellness*. Much of my work as a New Age coach is to orchestrate these arts.

I am including several self-report systems used by the Wholistic Health and Nutrition Institute of Mill Valley, with which I have been in affiliation for several years. There is also an excerpt from the health history used at Meadowlark, a Holistic Health Center in Hemet, California, founded 20 years ago by the visionary homeopathic doctor and surgeon, Dr. Evarts Loomis.

Assessing your lifestyle will help you get to discover your *ignition switches*, the things that turn you on, hang-ups about your body and things you may never have seriously considered such as the way you use food, your values, and priorities. In a later chapter I will help you assess yourself physically and find out about such things as your structural alignment, the way you move in relation to gravity, and your overall flexibility.

You may be surprised at how little attention you have paid to the natural elements of a well-balanced life, or the skills you have left undeveloped, or the gifts neglected. You may be very surprised at how little you have *moved* over the past months or what percentage of your diet is *junk food* either from vending machines or fast food restaurants.

And you will probably be astounded at some of the "connections that click"; connections that allow you to begin and end your day with the smell of cut grass and flowers in your psyche. Perhaps your training program will include time to run and play with your children freely and joyously in the woods, a stretch on the living room floor instead of watching television, or a gravitation to natural health food stores rather than supermarkets. I hope that through awareness, reflection, and inspiration, you will find yourself on the new horizon of well-being.

Lifestyle Review

The first step in your Lifestyle Review is personally to evaluate your attitudes, habits, health history, personality functioning, and intuitive reflection.

I always begin my coaching sessions with a consultation in an aesthetic environment which is intimate and free of distractions. This promotes inspiration and reflection. Often I light candles, and put on soothing music to tune into the right hemisphere of the brain and bring out the subtleties of my client's life. I want to inspire a sense of trust in uniqueness, authenticity, a person's sense of inner wisdom, from which a training program can naturally flow. It is impossible to standardize a self-report system. When I allow people to reflect on their lives, I find that they organize their internal system of functioning and that a master plan dictates itself. I need only intercede occasionally to keep thoughts flowing.

I would suggest the following process for your Lifestyle Review and Personal Assessment. Begin with a block of time: at least two hours. Create an inspirational atmosphere, perhaps with a fire, music, candles. Take the phone off the hook and make sure there will be no distractions. Adopt the attitude that you are *painting a biographical portrait* for someone who doesn't know you. In painting the portrait you will sharpen colors and texture to allow richness in tone and aesthetic clarity to emerge.

Start talking into a tape recorder. Perhaps a friend or lover will sit with you and give you energy just *listening*. Their presence may assist you in bringing out the depth and clarity of your feelings. Do not start this review if you are under any emotional stress: anger, jealousy, trauma. Be honest about your positives and negatives as you follow the questions in each of the sections. Practice *free association*. Get both halves of your brain working: your left, which will see each question with a specific answer, and your right, which will provoke feelings. It is the weaving together of the two modes that you want to record and reflect on.

There are three approaches to choose from in conducting your Lifestyle Review: 1. A stream of consciousness in which you just relax and use the questions in this chapter to stimulate your thoughts. 2. A dialogue with another person based on the questions in this chapter. 3. A question and answer session in which you actually write out the answers to the questions.

A Combination

My preference is for a combination of the approaches. Begin by reviewing the material in this chapter on Lifestyle Review. Use the questions to conduct a stream of consciousness session with yourself. Wait a few days. Then go back and conduct either a dialogue or question and answer session. See what surfaces. Listen to the tapes of yourself before going to bed. Be sure to record your dreams that night. Keep a pencil and paper beside your bed. Be sure to have either a tape recorder or notepaper with you the next day for additional insights that will surface. Remember, you are training your total being, not just your physical body.

Questions for Lifestyle Review

In this section I am including a series of questions that you can use as a point of departure for your own Lifestyle Review.

Daily Schedule

1. What time of day do I get up? How long does it take for breakfast, to get dressed, to get to work, to get the children off to school?
2. If I arise 30 to 40 minutes earlier, what time would I have to go to bed in order to feel rested? What organization would it take?
3. What *significant others* are involved? Could they be included and how? What would it take?
4. What is my schedule like at lunch? Could I take a two hour break and get some physical activity one or two times a week?
5. Where is a park, pool, gym, place to run?
6. Could I use a stationary bike, do stretches, jump rope?
7. How could I sponge off, shower, change afterwards? At work, can shower facilities be installed?
8. At work, could we acquire some equipment: small trampoline, stationary bike, jump ropes, slant boards, weights, special exercise room?
9. If at home during day, how much time do I have completely to myself? When do I experience a slump in energy?

Evenings

1. How have I spent my evening hours for the last three weeks?
2. Do I overeat or drink too much due to stress and fatigue?
3. What interests have I failed to pursue because of tiredness?
4. How much time have I spent watching television because it's an easy out? Is it satisfying?
5. What time do I go to bed? How much sleep do I get? Quality?
6. Ask yourself honestly: "What am I doing that I feel is a waste of time?"

Environment

Reflect upon the stimulation you are receiving from your environment during the day.

1. Am I satisfied with the stimulation I am receiving from my environment? Do I feel comfortable at home? at my office? in my car?
2. When I come home, do I feel uplifted and calm? Am I refreshed?
3. If not, why? Is there too much clutter? Do I put off "getting things in order" because it exhausts me?
4. Are the people I live with truly conducive to my growth or are they damaging? Do I purposely get involved in *going out* to avoid unsatisfactory relationships with people at home?
5. What can I do to rectify my home or working environment so that my day is devoted to joy, productive living, and so that I can have a regular training program?
6. Am I procrastinating in regard to major life changes: job, school, marriage, love-life? Do I realize that it may require courage to alter my environment, to advance to the next level of my personal growth?
7. What would I like my environment to look and feel like? What do I have to do to bring about changes? Reflect and paint a picture.

View of Life Index

The *View of Life Index* can help you to reflect on how much *you* determine your reality. How do you experience your life? To what extent do you find meaning and purpose in your life? The *View of Life* questionnaire provides a mirror to help you reflect the reality you have created for yourself. You are the *owner* and *creator* of your view of your life. How much of your viewpoint is your own and how much has come from other people's point of view? How much of your life is *inner directed*? Who are you living your life for? Are you frustrated, bored? The answers to these simple questions may profoundly influence your experience of life and your state of health and may point to qualities of character you need to take into consideration when devising a Lifestyle Training Program.

For each of the following questions, rate yourself on a scale of 1 to 7, with 4 being neutral (no judgment at all).

Vitality

1. I am usually
   (1) completely bored
   (7) exuberant, enthusiastic
2. Life to me seems:
   (7) always exciting
   (1) completely boring
3. Facing my daily tasks is:
   (7) source of pleasure and satisfaction
   (1) painful, boring

4. Every day is:
   (7) constantly new and different
   (1) exactly the same
5 After retiring I would:
   (7) do some of the exciting things I have always wanted to
   (1) loaf completely the rest of my life

Life Goals

6. I have discovered:
   (1) no mission or purpose in life
   (7) clear-cut goals and a satisfying life purpose
7. In life I have:
   (1) no goals or aims
   (7) very clear goals and aims
8. In achieving life goals I have:
   (1) made no progress
   (7) progressed to complete fulfillment

Compatibility/Responsibility

9. As I view the world in relation to my life, the world:
   (1) completely confuses me
   (7) fits meaningfully with my life
10. I am a:
    (1) very irresponsible person
    (7) very responsible person

Personal Existence

11. My personal existence is:
    (1) utterly meaningless
    (7) very purposeful, full of meaning
12. In thinking of my life, I:
    (1) often wonder why I exist
    (7) always see a reason for my being here
13. If I could choose, I would:
    (1) prefer never to have been born
    (7) like nine lives just like this

14. My life is:

    (1) empty, filled with despair

    (7) running over with exciting good things

15. If I should die today, I would feel that my life has been:

    (7) very worthwhile

    (1) completely worthless

16. I regard my ability to find a meaning, purpose or mission in life as:

    (7) very great

    (1) practically none

Self Determination (Control)

17. Concerning man's freedom to make his own choices, I believe man is:

    (7) absolutely free to make all life choices

    (1) completely bound by limitations of heredity and environment

18. My life is:

    (7) in my hands and I am in control of it

    (1) out of my hands and controlled by external factors

Passage

19. With regard to death, I am:

    (7) prepared and unafraid

    (1) unprepared and frightened

Job

20. I experience my job as:

    (1) a drudgery, means to an end

    (7) great source of satisfaction, all I could hope for

21. My working relationship with my boss and/or peers is:

    (1) a constant source of anxiety and frustration

    (7) an absolute joy

22. My working conditions are:

    (7) exceptionally pleasant and comfortable

    (1) exceptionally distracting and uncomfortable

23. My income is:

    (7) adequately compensated, no complaint

    (1) a source of great anxiety, totally inadequate

Filling the Mind

The thoughts you hold in your mind, the degree of positive thinking, are also important. There is *innerspace* training that can propel you toward your life goals and a more joyous life. The first step is to reflect on these general questions concerning how you are now *filling up your mind.*

1. What am I doing now to inspire myself to my highest character aspirations? What do I read, listen to, see visually that stimulates my senses?

2. What books did I read last year? What did they mean to me? How did they inspire and ignite me to a fuller, more productive and joyous life? What books do I want to read?

3. What other things do I read? Magazines? Newspapers? What would I like to subscribe to?

4. What movies do I go to? Plays? Art shows? Entertainment? What effect do these have in *filling up my mind*?

5. What would I like to be stimulated by but am not?

6. What am I filling up my mind with that I honestly feel is a *waste of time*?

7. How much do I watch television? (Assess the last three weeks.) How much does television elevate me? Depress me? Is it just escapism and a waste of my life-force?

8. What do I wish I was doing instead of watching television? What do I think it would take for me to reorganize my life and do these other things? What changes would it make in my home environment?

9. How much time do I spend reading or viewing material that inspires my highest ideals of personal growth or gives me a sense of the joy of life?

10. How could *moments of beauty* or *inspirational breaks* be introduced into my life in place of *coffee breaks*? Reflect on the stimulation of your environment during the day and the effect it has on you; either energizing or depleting your energy. Make small lists of things you can do to make the situation be conducive to health. Be aware that stress from noise, smoke-filled areas, loud music, over-lighted rooms, driving through heavy traffic all affect what goes into your mind. Consider what specific small books or pamphlets, poetry, philosophy, art works, music could be in your environment and fill your mind with beauty, inspiration, and compassion.

Assessing Your Environment and Resources

1. What resources are available in my community for use in my training program? Is there a local track, gym, school, Y, community club?

2. Where are the health clubs or classes I could take? Where are they located? What do they cost? Would they fit into my schedule?

3. Where are the swimming pools, bike trails, stretches of soft dirt for running?

4. What *blueprint of resources* in my community could I put together to help me enjoy and stay on a training program?

5. What activities could I initiate among my circle of friends to motivate me toward physical activity either at home or work?

6. What equipment could I acquire for my home or office to facilitate a training program? Set of weights, slant board, small trampoline, jump rope?

7. Where could I go to use such equipment? How much does it cost? When could I realistically use it? What factors would I have to consider if I wanted to purchase some equipment?

8. What is obvious in my environment that I could use? Stairs, places to hang, running to and from work, parking the car one to three miles away and walking the rest?

9. Where could I put a mat to stretch or do yoga during the day?

10. If I travel, could I get rooms on the 7th floor (or higher) and run up and down stairs? Or where a pool or park is nearby?

11. How could I put a flexible program together to deal with sudden changes or emergencies and not fall behind in my training?

Health History

When I first went to Meadowlark, a holistic health center in Hemet, California, I had not been evaluated by a doctor who practiced from the viewpoint of *healing the whole person*. Dr. Evarts Loomis is such a doctor. Over many years, he has evolved a *Health History Questionnaire* and I found it so stimulating that I requested permission to use portions of it in this section. I now use this questionnaire with my clients to enhance their self-reflection. A few have sought guidance from practitioners of this discipline. Others have taken the information to their physicians. I encourage you to add this type of information to the insights you are gaining about your past, present and future and to take charge of guiding your own health care.

Head

1. Do you get headaches? What part of head hurts? What time of day?

2. Best description: Aching, boring.

3. What is the spread of location of the headache?

Sleep

1. How is your sleep?
2. Are you able to sleep in any position?
3. Do you feel refreshed after sleep?

Aches and Pains

1. Do you have any trouble in your back?
2. Is stiffness present?

Sexual Sphere

1. Is your sexual life satisfying to you?

Previous History

1. State all major illnesses suffered, such as malaria, typhoid, etc., with approximate dates and duration, whether you regained your health completely.

2. Have you recently become: doubtful, impatient, irritable, depressed, jealous, shy, restless, silent or talkative?

Previous Treatment

1. State all the medicines and treatments you have taken so far and the results.

Family History

1. State age and condition of health of the following. If not alive state age at and cause of death: Mother, Father, Brothers, Sisters, Spouse.

Life Change Index

This list, devised by Dr. Thomas H. Holmes of the University of Washington, shows the scale impact for each life change event. And, of course, the point to such a chart is not trying to come up with an absolute score for you but rather to get some idea of the relative amounts of stress triggered by different events.

100	Death of Spouse
73	Divorce
65	Marital Separation or end of love relationship
63	Jail Term
63	Death of close family member
53	Personal injury or illness / miscarriage / abortion

50 Marriage
47 Fired at Work
45 Marital/love relationship reconciliation
45 Retirement
44 Change in health of family member
40 Pregnancy
39 Sex Difficulties
39 Gain of new family member
39 Business readjustment
38 Change in financial state
37 Death of close friend
36 Change to different line of work
36 Change in number of arguments with spouse
31 Mortgage over $10,000
30 Foreclosure of mortgage or loan
29 Change in responsibilities at work
29 Son or daughter leaving home
29 Trouble with in-laws
28 Outstanding personal achievement
26 Spouse begins or stops work
26 Begin or end school
25 Change in living conditions
24 Revision of personal habits
23 Trouble with boss
20 Change in work hours or conditions
20 Change in residence
20 Change in schools
19 Change in recreation
19 Change in church activities
18 Change in social activities
17 Mortgage or loan less than $l0,000
16 Change in sleeping habits
15 Change in number of family get-togethers
15 Change in eating habits
13 Vacation (if approaching or on your mind)
12 Christmas (if approaching or on your mind)
11 Minor violations of the law

Nutrition

Food consciousness is a very important tool that can help us become aware of the many variables we must cope with in our hazardous industrial society. Food consciouness involves educating yourself about nutrition, being alert as to *risk* foods, being nutritionally aware with your family, making responsible food choices, and, most definitely, practicing what you preach.

The Eating Habits Survey is the finest self-analysis tool I've discovered to help you gain insights into what you're eating, why, your attitude towards food and over-all food consciousness. In Chapter 7, on Nutrition for the New Age, I outline general principles for proper nutrition. This is especially important since you will be using your body more strenuously on a training program and your food habits will change.

In responding to the Eating Habits Survey, be reflective. If examples or incidents come into your mind, allow them to flow onto the tape recorder. Be honest with yourself and genuinely reflect on your attitude towards food and the emotional or psychological needs it fills in your life.

Most of my clients on training programs undergo intensive nutritional analysis either by computer analysis based upon a hair sample or urine analysis. For purposes of this section I am including the Nutritional Evaluation used by WHN (Wholistic Health and Nutrition Institute of Mill Valley) at the Nutri-Lab in Hayward, California. You can obtain information about your own profile directly. Remember that keeping track of what you eat and the supplements you take will help to enhance your training program.

Eating Habits Survey

For the statements below, express how frequently each occurs: very frequent, often, occasional, seldom, never.

1. Eat excessively when bored or depressed.
2. Insomnia.
3. Eat foods you know are "bad" for you.
4. Prefer eating alone.
5. Feel conspicuous or embarrassed when eating with others.
6. Parents used, had available, or encouraged sweets.
7. Fear weight gain.
8. "To hell with it all" feeling.
9. Will sneak or hide foods.
10. Alcoholic beverages.
11. Eat foods discouraged by your parents.
12. Eat or drink in secrecy.
13. Drugs (tranquilizers, sleeping pills, appetite suppressants, etc.)
14. Self-conscious of how my body looks.
15. Wish I looked different.
16. Feelings (diet or otherwise) of being "rushed" or sense of time urgency.
17. Waves of anger or hostility.

18. Feelings (diet or otherwise) of being in the midst of "struggle."
19. Fatigue or "wiped out" feelings.
20. Uncontrollable hunger urges.
21. Gulp your food.
22. Stuff yourself.
23. Cravings for sweets.
24. Eat when not hungry.
25. Eat and "run."
26. Cravings for sweets.
27. Meals or heavy snacks after 7 p.m.
28. Eat within an hour of retiring.
29. Eating binges.
30. Pastries, soft drinks, candy, ice cream, etc.
31. Processed meats (smoked ham, bologna, sausage, bacon, etc.)
32. Use canned or processed foods.
33. Use commercial seasonings (catsup, salts, etc.)
34. Sugar in tea, coffee, fruits, etc.
35. Use salted butter or margarine.
36. Fried foods.
37. Salty foods (chips, crackers, etc.).
38. Antacids.
39. Laxatives.
40. Alcohol.
41. Coffee, tea.
42. Instant Breakfast, Tang, Pop-tarts, etc.
43. Artificially flavored breakfast cereal.
44. Read and appreciate labels.
45. Raw fruits and vegetables.
46. Vitamin supplements.
47. Try to eat a balanced diet.
48. Drink 8 glasses of water or liquid equivalent daily.
49. Nutritionally aware with your family.
50. Whole grains or whole grain bread.
51. Use of herbs — fresh or dried.
52. Wheat germ, yeast, protein supplement.
53. Milk, eggs, cheese, or flesh foods.
54. Chew thoroughly.
55. Avoid "contrived" foods (insta-breakfasts, desserts, cereals, etc.).

56. Eat smaller more frequent meals.

57. Understand and avoid "hidden" sugars put in processed foods.

58. Read and educate yourself about nutrition.

59. Practice what you preach about good nutrition.

60. Understand and utilize "fasting."

61. Variety of fresh foods in daily diet.

62. When I am hungry, I usually prefer: green salad, fresh fruit, or pastry.

63. When I am thirsty, I usually prefer: fresh fruit juice or soda pop.

64. When I am hungry, I usually prefer: baked potato or french fries.

65. When I am hungry, I usually prefer: whole grain or white bread.

66. I use these foods for reward, escape, or punishment:

67. When I'm on a binge, my feelings before and after are:

68. In the former sections, which if any of the statements were significant or revealing to you? Why?

69. What foods do you fear? Why?

Physical Activity

I have purposely save the Physical Activity section until the end. I wanted to show you some of the many other variables involved in a Lifestyle Training Program. You, like so many, have probably not considered that what you do with your body is connected to everything else you do. And you may be aware of the enormous contradictions to a *lifestyle of total health* in many so-called *athletes.* For example, think about a runner who trains five miles a day and downs cokes, french fries, coffee. Or, as I see so frequently, highly competitive athletes who are "sugar-holics" or dancers who smoke.

It's not that we have to cut out completely all our *bad habits* to follow the principles in this book. But my job as a New Age Coach is to call your attention to the parameters that are relevant to a training program that will benefit all of you: body, mind, and spirit!

1. How much and what kind of physical exercise have I had the last three weeks?

2. What has *turned me on* the most?

3. How often do I work up a sweat and exercise my cardiovascular system?

4. How often have I stretched my body and spinal column? How much?

5. What are five activities that I would enjoy doing and am not now

currently engaged in? Rate these activities from one to five in order of preference.

6. What would it take for me to do one or more of these activities? Join a club or health spa, take a class, rearrange my schedule, care for an old injury, lose weight?

7. What people and obligations would I have to consider to do these activities regularly?

8. What travel, expenses, daylight hours, weather conditions would I have to examine?

9. How have I spent the last three weekends, or three representative weekends? How much exercise did I get?

10. How much time do I spend in spectator or *escape* activity rather than in moving my body?

11. What do I eat and drink on weekends that may make me sluggish or lethargic? Which of these could I reduce or eliminate?

12. What am I interested in pursuing that might elevate my spirit and also inspire me to more physical exercise? A trip to the country, concerts, sports, games, massages, saunas, meditation groups, devotional services of my choosing?

13. How could my evenings and weekends be devoted to a lifestyle that would enhance my health, inner growth, enable me to get exercise, be with people, and participate in activities that inspire me?

Stevanne Becomes a Butterfly

I would like to close this chapter with a personal vignette of a rather remarkable woman whose story may be an inspiration to you. She, like Edward, the executive in Chapter 1, lived a one-dimensional life. Her training program was initiated through inspiration, self-assessment, and scheduling.

It was dawn at Asilomar beach near Carmel, California. I was conducting an early morning training and meditation with a group of important health planners drawn together to chart the course of national legislation and social policy. The light was quiet, our mood high, and I had suggested initiating the day with inspiration from nature. After stretches and a jaunt over the sand dunes, we did long slow distance training, interspersed with visualizations. We closed with interval and wind sprints. As the group was dispersing, Stevanne sidled next to me and said, "Dyveke, I really want to get my body together. Will you be my coach?" Later we played tennis and ended the day with three hours of dancing.

I visited her at her home for a consultation. She explained her busy schedule, reflected on the areas we have mentioned in this chapter, analyzed the stress in her life, and took a serious look at her time demands. She was obviously intelligent but had not previously analyzed the data we examined during the consultation. It was obvious that we needed to devise a program within the confines of her house and backyard, with two rest periods for meditation to "visualize the body she desired." I encouraged her to keep her initial program simple and manageable and not feel overwhelmed by another demand. I wrote up her *training schedule*. I even gave her a master session, jumping up and down steps and stretching as we strolled the streets of San Francisco en route to a sauna. I hoped to instill in her an attitude of playing with her environment.

Stevanne Auerbach at that time was so busy writing, researching, organizing, teaching, and mothering that she was sleeping only three or four hours a night. She is a nationally recognized child care expert who spends half her day on the phone arranging speaking engagements and conferences. Not only does she hold a doctorate, she has authored three books, and is in the forefront of the current cultural changes. The pace and depth of her activities inspired me to devise a unique training program for her.

When I visited her recently, she was crosslegged on a cushion on the floor of her cozy apartment. Her thick dark hair was flowing and she was wearing a bright blue blouse embroidered with a butterfly, a symbol that she loves and has just finished writing a book about.

> The sun is filtering through her lace curtains and she sips an herbal tea instead of the coffee and Danish she once would have needed in mid-morning. Butterfly motifs, gay tapestries, and a soft pastel charcoal portrait of her drawn by a friend decorate her walls.
>
> She's very different from the professionally active, physically inactive woman I first met on that beach at Asilomar, California. "When we went out for our first sessions, I didn't think I could run a half a block. I had never run before. But I went out on that beach and just started doing it with you and those doctors. *I felt like a toad, like a baby elephant.* I saw you as a strong, powerful, dynamic woman who had her body under control and felt comfortable coming from a physical place. I had my PhD. My intellectual gifts were well in hand, but not my body. I guess you inspired me also because you were older and made me feel youthful. It made me feel that if I could get my body into shape I could do anything. That was the ignition switch: the inspiration that changed my picture of myself.
>
> "The butterfly has been an important symbol for me. It has symbolized my own metamorphosis and change. I have experienced spiritual connections to nature, to ecology, to the environment, to the problems of butterflies becoming extinct. They are so beautiful and so fragile. The fragileness in nature is in ourselves. They are a symbol to me of people going through transformation. What's happened to me is that I've gone through being a lumpy caterpillar and into a period of incubation. I'm visualizing myself as very thin. I will lose all of the excess fat, all of the heaviness of spirit. Before, I took the problems of the kids very seriously. I took child care very seriously. I have been heavy. What I want to do is lighten up. I'm becoming the butterfly I want to be."

Two years have passed since Stevanne and I met on that beach. I asked her to share what her training has meant to her and what she could share with others. Not having seen her for almost a year, the first thing I noticed was the *spring and bounce and light-footedness with which she moved.* I exclaimed: "Stevanne, you move like a real athlete." Indeed, her lifestyle has changed.

> The training gave me a new way to move. It gave me a new picture of myself. I see myself for the first time as a *dancer in flight.* I was smoking two packs of cigarettes a day, didn't see myself as a writer, drank, and was 25 pounds overweight. I generally felt low and this low self-esteem was manifested in my body. In these two years the smoking and alcohol have stopped and my diet is basically vegetarian. I do yoga 25 minutes a day and run at least four mornings a week. I run up to five miles. My sex life and my total energy have improved. Now I see myself as something light, beautiful and colorful. You gave me your favorite scarf. I've worn it ever since. I feel like a transformed butterfly.

Prelude to
I Will Change
My Life

It is midnight. I have been working on my book all day. My schedule calls for me to be back at 6:30 a.m. I have a light snack of nuts, seeds, and a piece of fruit. As I lie down on my bed, I take a deep breath, filling my abdomen with air. Then I blow out an image of the number one, stored deep within my abdomen; out through the wall, across the Tufts Athletic Field, toward the Prudential building several miles away in Boston. Then I pull it all the way back across the field, through the wall and deep into my abdomen. I repeat this process several times and begin to feel very relaxed.

As I lie there in the space between waking and sleeping realities, I let my mind drift through Roberto Assagioli's book *The Act of Will*. Back come the thoughts of a time when my life fell apart. It was then that I took Assagioli's theory into my own body, life, and psyche. And from out of my own life's experiences, I have developed techniques for systematically training the will. I want to communicate these in my writing. My consciousness is saturated with thoughts on training the will. I drift into a quiet sleep.

Throughout the night, I dream. As I awake in the morning, five minutes before the alarm goes off, I am aware that I dreamed but can't recall the specific details. I do know that my ideas on training the will were woven into each dream in some way.

I have planned to run to the office, three miles away, this March morning. It is very cold, about 25 degrees, with a stiff wind that will be blowing against me as I run. Though it is warm and cozy in the bed I have no trouble getting up and putting on my running clothes. It is as if nature were beckoning to me to come out and be a part of its majesty and beauty.

41

After doing my regular 30-minute routine of stretching exercises, I step out the door. My trail will be the bare pavement of Massachusetts streets between four-foot snowdrifts; not even the luxury of sidewalks. I will be struggling with the cars and buses carrying early morning commuters. I think how essential training of the will is to those who must face these environmental conditions every day during the winter.

As I run, I think, "What was it that got me out here this morning in the cold and wind? I didn't 'force' myself to do my training. I was *inspired* by the trees and the sky. They beckoned to me and their invitation filled my heart with a desire to be a part of that *something bigger* outside. My environment had stimulated and excited my inner drive, to mobilize and direct my energy (my *will*) to have a morning run. When I was a student at the conservatory, I always wondered what it was about a piece of music that could so excite my imagination that I was willing to put in literally hundreds of hours of practice. I always questioned why one did it and another didn't. I realized it was that sense of *inner inspiration*, that *ignition switch* And this is what I felt, gazing at the trees and sky and feeling the exhilaration that would occur soon as my cheeks would burn, sweat would freeze around my ears, and the sound of the crisp ice would make me feel alive.

As I run, I feel connected to the men and women who pioneered a new nation and grappled with the elements of snow and cold each year without modern conveniences. I am inspired by their courage and fortitude. I also think of the thousands of people to whom I will be speaking in my book. I am suddenly conscious that, for many of these people, this book will represent a perspective and perhaps a formula to get their lives together; to discover their inner beauty, to begin the pursuit of their wildest dream. I find myself praying to the universe to allow me to be a channel through which this message can flow. I am very aware of my humanity.

During the last third of my run, the outline of the chapter forms in my mind. It is as if the pre-sleep meditation, my dreams, and my run have served as a warmup for the actual writing, just as stretching exercises serve as a warmup for my runs. As I sit down in front of my desk, I realize that this whole experience has been an exercise in training my will.

Chapter Three:
I Will Change
My Life

Assessing Your Will

When you begin a physical training program you will be beseiged by hidden monsters in your psyche. These monsters can be likened to *secret sirens* deflecting you from the path of your *ego ideal*: a healthy, radiant, fit body. You will find every excuse in the world not to get out of bed. You may be under tremendous stress at work and just not have it in you to "go out there and face it today." A spat with a lover or spouse, errands to do, bad weather, aching shoulders . . . all these nagging urges can deter you from getting started and staying on a training program.

What you are facing is your *will*, a silent inner power that is operating all the time.

As a New Age Coach I soon discovered that *training the will* is the single most important element in laying the base for a training program. For a long time I couldn't understand why people who wanted to improve their lives and were reasonably together would continue to perform such destructive acts, negating their fullest potentials, culminating in stress. Each day in my consultations and coaching sessions, repeatedly in workshops, the theme recurred, "I know I've got to get on a training program. I really want to but I just don't seem to have the willpower. I'm not disciplined enough."

It was not until I discovered that *training the will* is a science, as well as an art form, that I saw its relevance to helping others. At this time my person-

43

al life had fallen apart. The ideas and teaching of Dr. Roberto Assagioli and Psychosynthesis were a key factor in helping me get my life together and proceed with my work. The training of the will not only helped resurrect my own life but laid the conceptual base for my profession as New Age Coach.

In this chapter, I will condense and share the ideas from Assagioli's teachings and my own experiences, and show how they can be applied in lifestyle training.

> The discovery of the will in oneself, and the realization that the self and will are intimately connected, may come as a revelation that can change your self-awareness. You see yourself as a *living subject* endowed with the power to choose, to relate, to bring about changes in your personality, in others, in circumstances. This enhanced awareness, this awakening and vision of new, unlimited potentialities for inner expansion and outer action, gives a new feeling of confidence, security, joy; a sense of wholeness.
>
> But this initial revelation, this inner light, however vivid and inspiring at the moment of its occurrence, is apt to grow dim and flicker out. The new awareness of self is easily submerged by the constant surge of drives, desires, emotions, and ideas. It is crowded out by the ceaseless inrush of impressions from the outer world. Thus the need to protect, cultivate, strengthen the will to make it an enduring possession and utilize its great possibilities.
>
> We all have a tendency towards inertia. We let the "easygoing" side of our nature take control, allowing inner impulses or external influences to dominate our personality. It may be summed up as unwillingness to "take the trouble," to pay the price demanded by a worthwhile undertaking. (*The Act of Will*, pp 9-11)

Thus, beginning a training program is a new voyage on which you can start to realize you are a human being with a will that must be trained along with your physical body through the powers of your mind.

Roberto Assagioli puts the will in perspective when he says that it is like the director of a play, marshalling all the available resources to accomplish a specific purpose. The function of the will is often misconstrued as applying force towards one's personality as a dictator. It is impossible to become ignited and reorganize your lifestyle so that you may begin and stay on a training program, without simultaneously training your will. So first it is important for you to know what the will is, how important it can be in facilitating your life's goals, and how to systematically discipline your inner resources so that you are propelled effortlessly and lovingly towards your most cherished dreams.

The will in action has a number of characteristics:
1. Energy-Dynamic Power-Intensity
2. Mastery-Control-Discipline
3. Concentration-One-Pointedness-Attention-Focus
4. Determination-Decisiveness-Resoluteness-Promptness

5. Initiative-Courage-Daring
6. Organization-Integration-Synthesis

Each of us has modes of functioning that strengthen some of these characteristics. Other qualities need "tooling up" and your training program can be used to build strength in your weak areas.

Assagioli talks about the four aspects of the will: the strong will, the good will, the skillful will and the transpersonal will. Often the strong will is not enough. The skillful use of the will is required to overcome barriers that would ordinarily stop a person who has a certain strength of will. We will see later in this chapter how Linda was able to train her will in a skillful way that enabled her to continue a stalled training program. She actually strengthened her will by conducting activities that increased her motivation.

The fourth aspect of the will, the transpersonal will, deals with that part of life which is "beyond oneself." It concerns the embracing of all living things in both the animal and vegetable kingdoms. It involves a sense of spiritual unity, of life as a mystery, of the oneness and interconnectedness of things.

In this section, I want you to make an assessment of your own will both in terms of the four aspects of the will described above and in terms of Assogioli's six phases of the act of willing. Assogioli describes the process of willing as:

1. Determination of your goals. You must decide which goals you want to pursue. There are many things we want to do in life from the very important to the trivial. We need to make our goals explicit.

2. Determining the priority of your goals. This involves deliberaton. This is the step of deciding the relative importance of your goals.

3. Choosing a goal to pursue and setting aside or discarding others. We often let trivial goals get in the way of pursuing our key goals. We have to learn to put first things first.

4. Affirming that what is willed shall happen. This involves the technique of acting *as if* what is willed has already happened. See in your mind's eye a picture of the goal as accomplished. In essence this means retaining it unswervingly in your mind and not letting the vision of the final accomplishment get lost in the means of accomplishing it.

5. Formulating a plan that consists only of the essential means for realizing the plan and determining that the plan is feasible, flexible, and is pursued with a cooperative spirit toward others involved.

6. The direction of the materials, energies, and means toward the execution of the plan.

As Assagioli points out, these six functions are not all of equal importance in every decision. And only important decisions warrant a formal application of the functions. But it is important to assess how well you perform each one of the functions and that you employ training exercises to improve the functions on which you are weak. If you fail to reach a goal you can be sure that it is because you failed adequately to complete one of the six functions.

Exercises for Strengthening the Will

Realizing the Value of the Will

Settle yourself into a comfortable position with your muscles relaxed.

A. Picture to yourself as vividly as possible the loss of opportunity, the damage, the pain to yourself and others which has actually occurred, and which might again occur, as a result of the present lack of strength of your will. Examine these occasions, one by one, formulating them clearly; then make a list of them in writing. Allow the feelings which these recollections and forecasts arouse to affect you intensely. Then let them evoke in you a strong urge to change this condition.

B. Picture to yourself as vividly as possible all the *advantages* that an effective will can bring you; all the benefits, opportunities, and satisfactions which will come from it to you and others. Examine them carefully, one by one. Formulate them with clarity and write them down. Allow the feelings aroused by these anticipations to have full sway: the *joy* of the great possibilities that open up before you; the *intense desire* to realize them; the *strong urge* to begin at once.

C. Picture yourself vividly as being in possession of a strong will. See yourself walking with a firm and determined step, acting in every situation with decision, focused intention, and persistence. See yourself successfully resisting any attempt at intimidation and enticement. Visualize yourself as you will be when you have attained inner and outer mastery. (*The Act of Will* p. 36)

This exercise has endless uses: to reprogram faulty eating habits, instill the discipline necessary to continue a training program, to reprogram negative psychological functioning, e.g. the tendency to withdraw from situations that need confrontation, for fear of being criticized.

You can *evoke feelings towards the will* by using reading material to cultivate and reinforce your will. The material should be encouraging, positive, and dynamic in character to arouse self-reliance and incite to action. Biographies of outstanding personalities who have possessed great will are excellent to awaken your inner energies.

It is best not to talk about your activities to strengthen the will, or try to induce others to follow. *Work in silence*. Talking tends to dissipate the energies needed and accumulated for action. You don't want to provoke skeptical or cynical remarks as you *train your will and embark upon a training program*.

The gynmastics of the will can be trained by *useless exercises*. This approach consists of carrying out a number of simple and easy little tasks, with precision, regularity and persistence. Each task requires several days or a week and is replaced by another to avoid monotony. Muscles become stronger by a series of contractions. There are specific exercises that can be used to strengthen a weak part of the body. Similarly, to strengthen the will, it is best to exercise it independently of every other psychological function. This can be accomplished by performing deliberate acts which have no other purpose than the *training of the will*.

Useless Exercises to Train the Will

> Each day, for the next seven days, I will stand on a chair here in my room, for ten consecutive minutes, and I will try to do so contentedly. At the end of this ten-minute task write down the sensations and the mental states you have experienced during that time. Do the same on each of the seven days.
>
> Repeat quietly and aloud, "I *will* do *this*," keeping time with rhythmic movements of a stick or ruler for five minutes.
>
> Walk to and fro in a room, touching in turn, say, a clock on the mantelpiece and a particular pane of glass, for five minutes.
>
> Listen to the ticking of a clock or watch, making some definite movement at every fifth tick.
>
> Get up and down from a chair 30 times.
>
> Replace in a box, very slowly and deliberately, one hundred matches or bits of paper (an exercise particularly adapted to combat impulsiveness). (*The Act of Will* p. 40)

The Technique of Evocative Words

Certain words have a great effect on our moods and ideas. Such words as serenity, courage, joy, compassion are stimulating and arouse certain *feelings*. We can use evocative words to express the quality we want to evoke within ourselves. Put them on a card in a place easily noticed, especially near your bed, and look at it before sleep. Place several about your house or room. This might be called a *beneficent obsession*. Using the exercises mentioned before to strengthen the will, you can reflect upon the meaning of the word, feel the psychological quality the word embodies, say it aloud or write it several times.

Often when students are beginning a training program they will make scrolls with affirmations about what they desire. Put a large piece of paper the full length of your wall. Write in bold ink or crayon all of your desires and goals, whether to correct a habit or instill courage, or discipline your will to assist you to run four times a week. Give yourself a name, like *Courageous Charlie* or *Marathon Mary*. Identify with your new self-image. Place line after line all the things you want to to see happen. Use strong statements: "I, John, deeply desire and strongly am dedicated to . . . ''

There is hardly anyone I've worked with who hasn't found that systematically training the will through scrolls, affirmations, journals, cards with evocative words, useless exercises, or self-made training tapes with affirmations, has significantly facilitated their goals.

I am suggesting that we all need to train our wills in different ways. A type-A hard-driving executive may have a strong will and execute prodigous work output and be afraid to express feelings of negativity. He needs to train his will in compassion and expressiveness, and take the risk of being *rejected*. Others may have terrible feelings of self-worth and be shy about moving their bodies in public. Their wills need to be strengthened in hope, courage, grandeur. They may need to read books and articles about heroic people who have overcome great obstacles to resurrect their health, people such as Percy Wells Cerutty, the Master Olympic Coach, who was my teacher and inspirer.

Men and the Will

In my coaching I have found some differences between men and women in terms of the will. Most men have very highly developed wills. They get the data. They get the picture. They see the logic of a physical training program. They are very used to working against pressure and deadlines. They are used to coming up against adversity. The entire *masculine principle* is at their disposal. But without awakening the other, *being* values, the humane values of inner awareness, they will continue to train as automatons . . . totally out of touch with their feelings, totally masochistic and not developing all the available aspects of their personality. Sooner or later, only a few of the men who approach training in this way will be able to sustain a training program through all the obstacles of employment, family, friends, weather, etc. Most will falter.

Women and the Will

With most women the act of exercising the will is the exact opposite of that of men. Women may initially have a very hard time sticking to the discipline required to stay on a training program. For one thing, they have absolutely no cultural reinforcement because their bodies have been viewed as sex objects. They are surrounded by commercialism which makes them feel very inadequate and insecure. As a result they go out and buy extraneous trivia like the latest fashion, make-up, perfume . . . things to put on the outside of a seductive package, rather than training for *power from with-in.*

The nature of women is such that they are much more plugged in to that upper limit and the nature of the *transpersonal will* because they are the *mothers of the race.* They have an instinctive sense of protecting the seed force of the life that grows inside them, and to which they give birth. And they are linked through the *feminine principle* to feelings and intuitions. Women are much more naturally plugged into the transpersonal will, the sense of things beyond themselves.

When it comes to training the body, there is a natural instinct in women to be considered: women are more self-protective. Women find it harder to "play the upper limits" of their physicalness than do men. They don't like the sweat, cold, dirt, and inconveniences of physical training.

Women are relationship-oriented. Many women see their role and function as taking care of everyone else's needs first. For a woman to get on a regular systematic training program and see that her daily training is top priority, she must train the part of her will which values herself first. She must also overcome all the masochistic self-programming inside her psyche. This, in essence, is what Linda had to do. She utilized her skillful will to supplement the lack of strength in her will.

Linda

Linda had begun a Lifestyle Training Program but was having a terrible time continuing it because, as she said, "I felt so bad about my body that I didn't want anyone to see my fat jiggling around when I was running." After weeks of stops and starts, she decided that she needed to "get off the track and into my feelings." She needed to believe and trust in herself; to believe that her body would change, that she could discipline her thoughts and keep them positive. In short, she needed to train her will.

We experimented. For two weeks, she listened to a training tape which included positive affirmations such as "I desire to feel beautiful inside." "I know I have a responsibility to appreciate my life force and contribute my energies to the world in a constructive way."

We mobilized a nutritional workup and Linda changed her diet. On the training tapes, she visualized herself sitting at a meal with the appropriate natural foods. I composed music to inspire her and included that on the training tapes.

For weeks, she used the training tape and evoked the visualizations throughout the day, even while at work. She walked everywhere, once across the city of San Francisco for an appointment. She practiced the visualizations on the walk; even got a small pocket tape recorder to record her feelings. After two weeks, she started running again.

Meanwhile, she surrounded her house with affirmations about what she desired for herself. A beautiful scroll hung beside her bed with inspirational sayings, interspersed with poetry about the majesty of life. She began to work with the book *The Act of Will* by Roberto Assagioli.

When she resumed training, she took along a friend who was ten pounds more overweight than she was. Linda became her coach.

I had given Linda a total of three coaching sessions. She attended one workshop and designed one tape. We stayed in touch by telephone.

Linda had also agreed to keep a stream-of-consciousness journal of her changing attitudes, continue to work on her nutrition with a biochemist, get a few chiropractic adjustments, and have one or two acupuncture treatments. We discovered her pancreas was functioning sluggishly, causing digestive difficulties and some hypoglycemia (low blood sugar) which also contributed to her overweight condition.

All this took place in a matter of a few months, and Linda was totally in charge of directing and orchestrating the unfolding of her program.

I didn't see her again for six months. By then she was truly another woman. Her body tight and much slimmer. But what made me "shiver" was the beautiful inner light; the glow of inner beauty that radiated from her eyes. Not only had she *trained her will* in order to motivate herself, but she had inspired her friend to begin training. Now they have formed a small training group around their apartment complex.

Training the Skillful Will

In Chapter 2, you completed a Lifestyle Review which helped you to see not only who you *are* but who you *want to be*. In Chapters 4 and 5, we will provide you with information about how to use physical training and the feminine principle to help you to train your body to totally develop all aspects of your being; the physical as well as the mental and spiritual. Through this training of the whole person, you will become more and more in touch with your inner beauty, your feelings. You can't do this in a body that is polluted, toxified, and untrained. You will need to train your body to realize a higher meaning in life; to assume more and more of your rightful place in the universe.

This training will not always be easy. Just starting it may be one of the most difficult things you have ever attempted. And once started, you will need to apply the full powers of your will to keep it going. I have found, in the many years of my coaching, when a person gets ignited to start a training program, the critical moment comes when he or she must mobilize a schedule to do it and sustain that schedule through the ups and downs of the injuries and travails of life. You must *will* yourself to start and to continue your physical, mental, and spiritual training. And, as we have seen, you cannot rely on so-called "willpower." A strong will can help you but it is not sufficient in itself to bring you to the New Age ideal of being a totally developed, loving human being in body, mind, and spirit.

In the following sections, we will give some examples of exercises you can use for training the will.

Exercises to Strengthen the Skillful Will

1. *Substitution*: Withdrawing attention from a negative thought process can generate a positive feedback loop by substituting the qualities one desires by *visualizing and affirming a substitute*. Attention centered on any object gives it energy, making it more important to our awareness. Much of our inner clutter can be dealt with by the simple technique of substitution.

2. *Psychological breathing and freedom*: There are many harmful factors which pollute our psychological environment. These negative factors are aggressiveness and violence, fear, depression and despondency, greed and all forms of selfish desire. These poisons exist in our environnment and within ourselves. The most effective way to liberate positive energy is to *withdraw attention*. The act of this withdrawal of attention is an act of the skillful will, and in turn contributes to the strengthening of the will.

3. *Neutralization*: the active cultivation of qualities that are the antithesis of the harmful ones. i.e., harmlessness and nonviolence in the face of violence; courage in the place of fear; joy in healthy pleasures instead of depression; true love instead of consumptive sexuality.

4. *Acting As If* Techniques: Acting or behaving with the intention of manifesting qualities and states of being that we desire; when we act in this manner, such behavior actually changes our emotional states. By consciously adopting an attitude or action, the corresponding emotions and feelings will change. This is one of the most powerful tools to train the skillful will.

> When it is necessary or desired to overcome strong adverse tendencies or emotions, fear for instance, it is frequently helpful to precede the "acting as if" technique with that of the "ideal model." This entails visualizing ourselves as we would want to become, seeing ourselves in imagination acting in the manner in which we would like to act in actual practice. (*The Act of Will* pp 66-84)

Changing Your Environment

In all "recipe books" on physical training, little is said about the problems of motivation. One expert on physical fitness and nutrition, Chuck Richardson, says "Even in the finest cardiac-rehabilitions centers where the doctors say, 'Hey buddy, if you don't exercise, your next heart attack is *it*,' the attrition rate is still 70 percent."

We don't do what we should do solely out of fear, threat of failure, or even death. We do what we want to do because it is fun, enjoyable, interesting, inspirational. I have always believed this and this is why all my work is based upon motivating by inspiration. All I'm saying is that we live in such an incredibly beautiful world, in such an incredible biochemical machine, that we can't help but be inspired or take a day of life for granted. But I do and you do. We have to work every day on inspiring ourselves and believing that the world needs our sometimes seemingly small human gifts of energy. Each day we need to reawaken our sense of awe at the sheer miracle of being alive.

One of the best exercises for training your will is to provide yourself with a beautiful, aesthetic, inspirational environment. Surround yourself with beauty. Use your commuting time in cars or buses to listen to beautiful music or evocative phrases that you have taped. Try to get your employer to alter your work environment so that you feel uplifted every time you go to work. Bring beauty, music, poetry, love into your apartment or house.

Creating Positive Emotional States

As you begin to perform the rituals and exercises of training the will, you will find that your negative emotional states state to become positive. For example, if you have a hard time getting started on your training in the morning, you might proceed as Fred does and put on some Beethoven, read a poem, or think some loving thoughts toward someone that you are having a fight with. You will find that this will help you go out into the cold and run on the snow and pavement with a sense of joy. It isn't nearly as difficult now because your mind is filled with other thoughts; thoughts more joyous and elevated.

As you implement these exercises and learn to touch the inner state of joy, you will find that within three to four weeks you are easily able to get out of bed, get on your training clothes, and face the outside environment with a sense of expectation and joy; whether the environment is a warm California day or a cold, raw New England day. When you come back from your run you will feel an inner sense of beauty.

Igniting the Transpersonal Will

One of the most important parts of training the will is learning to feel an inner sense of beauty and to rise above the limitations of present reality. This is what the other end of the training spectrum is all about. I want to give you tools that you can use to evoke moments of personal transcendence regularly rather than randomly and accidentally. This is called training the transpersonal will. The transpersonal will has to do with getting a sense of the spiritual unity of life; ultimate values, higher needs, ecstasy, mystical experience, transcendence of the self. This is the domain concerned with the meaning of life.

We all have a need to understand the meaning of life. We all have times of crises, sense of personal futility. An individual feels that he or she is useless, life has no point or value and can lead nowhere. We need to reaffirm our *will to meaning*. We need to face courageously and willingly the requirements for transcending the limitations of personal consciousness without losing the center of individual awareness. Sudden, unexpected illumination without any previous conscious striving or exertion is a pull from the transpersonal self.

In my lectures, workshops, and private coaching, what sets me apart as a New Age Coach is that I am *consciously attempting to inspire and ignite the transpersonal will*. I use artistic creativity to awaken altruistic and humanitarian impulses, for these inspirations and urges goad an individual to assume undertakings and take actions that are *beyond* current functioning. The following example, written by one of my students, illustrates the process that ignited his transpersonal will:

> The first time I saw Dyveke was on a beautiful Sunday morning in October of 1977. I was attending the 1977 Holistic Health Conference at the Harvard Science Center in Cambridge, Massachusetts. There was to be a talk on fitness by Dyveke Spino. I was really excited about this because my life was being radically changed by work I was doing with my body. The previous speakers had dwelled on the mind and how the mind can alter bodily processes. I had spent all summer and fall studying and practicing meditation and relaxation and I was learning how powerful the mind is. But my entry point into these New Age ideas was from the body. I was amazed at how the *body* can affect the mind.
>
> I was also a little puzzled that many of the people I knew who were interested in New Age ideas had bodies that were in shambles. Many of them smoked, were overweight, never exercised. They spent a lot of time meditating and practicing spiritual healing but seemed to have no appreciation of how their bodies were deteriorating.
>
> Until the previous April, I had been the most sedentary of people. I didn't smoke, drink, or eat sugar, but I also never walked when I could ride, and never ran when I could walk. One Saturday, a year earlier, I walked the four miles from Harvard Square in Cambridge, Massachusetts to my home in Arlington. The last mile was torture. I was really wiped out in the evening.
>
> But then, in April of 1977, I started a course called psychoenergetics which was largely composed of deep breathing exercises. Two weeks after starting the course, I found my body literally begging me to do some of the exercises at home. Before I knew it I was spending nearly an hour and a half a day with these exercises, followed by a half hour of meditation and relaxation.
>
> Then one day I decided I should do some running. I had run for a few months ten or so years ago. But at the time I didn't know what I was doing, and severely injured my knees. I had never enjoyed running. I liked its effects but I hated the thought of getting out to run. And during the run

I was always in agony, doing anything I could in my mind to ease the mental and physical pain. The only good part was the shower at the end.

I started to run in September. I ran a mile the first night. Then I worked up to a mile of running, a half-mile of walking and a final half-mile of running. I immediately started to feel better but I still hated the thought of running. I bought a book on jogging, hoping that it would tell me how jogging could be fun. I read it and got some interesting information, but none that changed my attitude.

This was my orientation as I waited to hear Dyveke speak. I considered this to be my last chance to find a way to make jogging fun. I had no idea that there would be a radical change in my whole lifestyle: my approach to fitness, to nutrition, to my environment and to aesthetics.

At about 10:30 Dyveke bounded onto the stage. Her body was obviously powerful but at the same time sensuous. Her voice was exciting and soothing at the same time. Her effect on the audience was electric. She captured our imagination with her first few words. We were completely tuned in.

As she talked, it was as if I was being hit with a huge shot of adrenaline. She was saying how important it was to lay a physical base. She was talking about cardiovascular work, stretching, moving with different gaits. But she was also talking about visualizing, meditating, becoming one with the universe; all in the context of extending the limits of the body and the mind. And it hit me: this woman is putting it all together. She isn't just talking about the mind or the body, she's talking about the interaction between the two from both directions. This was the theoretical basis that I had been searching for: one that gave the body its rightful place and yet emphasized the full powers of the mind.

Then the movie screen came alive with a film of Percy Cerutty running with supreme grace, beauty, and energy. Dyveke was narrating. "This is Percy Cerutty, a man who, at the age of 45, with one lung and fused vertebrae, was given up for dead. He went out into the wilds of Australia and completely remade himself. He started to run, to grow his own food. He went on to coach some world-famous athletes who set many world records in speed and endurance: Herb Elliot, John Landy, Bill Emmerton."

As I watched the film, I was conscious that I was 40 years old. Many of the people I know who are in their 50s are beginning to go downhill physically. Many I know who are in their 60s have some trouble getting around, their bones are brittle, they have problems with stairs. I had given myself about 10 more years of active living. After that I believed the deterioration would set in. As I watched this man move, a sudden flash of insight exploded in my mind. I saw myself at the age of 80, with the same incredible grace and energy as this Percy Cerutty. I could hardly contain myself. I had just gained 40 more years of active, energetic, alive living.

I couldn't believe this was happening. The whole conference had been really exciting up to this point, but mainly from the standpoint of the the mind. This presentation was changing my whole life, in all its many facets, as I sat there.

Now Dyveke was telling us to stand up. We were going to do a little stretching; going to get some oxygen into our systems. She had us spread our legs and stretch over to the right. There we were 300 people of all shapes, sizes, conditions, standing between rows of stationary seats, trying to find room to move our bodies. We were completely connected to her.

Then Dyveke was showing a color film of her work. In the film, a group of women were running around in an amphitheater. It wasn't like any running I had ever seen. To me running was feet pounding on asphalt, arms high, shoulders locked, face grim and grimaced, racing against a partner and/or a stop watch, body shot full of pain. These women were so loose. Their gaits changed periodically from synchronous to asynchronous. At one point they gathered around a big rock and began a beautiful meditation about a sun star permeating each body, about each person's sun star being connected.

My mind was completely alive, completely attuned to the message of what I was later to know as the *feminine principle*. All I knew at this point was that my running would never be the same. I couldn't see all the implications but I somehow knew that running wasn't an end in itself. There was something about being connected to nature, about changing enviroments, bringing beauty into one's life, releasing the poetic and the heroic which all too often has been buried so deeply within us that we've forgotten it ever existed. There was something about the terrible price we've paid to become adults; about how we've left behind our imagination, stripped our lives of the aesthetic, downgraded our intuition in favor of statistics, proof, and logic.

There was something about how we're polluting our bodies with sugar, cigarettes, alcohol, processed foods; the temple of the spirit being defiled. But it doesn't have to be this way. There is a way out. And Dyveke was igniting us to dream our wildest dreams: about our bodies, our nutrition, our environment, our mind, and our spirit.

Now it was over and my body was trembling with emotion. I felt a return of childlike faith, innocence, imagination; I, who pride myself an organized and logical approach to problem-solving, could allow my feelings, my intuition an equal status in my life with my logic. I, who have abused my body for 40 years, could be an *athlete in training*. I, who have valued efficiency and work over beauty, can have both without feeling guilty. I can change the sterile environment of my employees into a work atmosphere that will lift their and my spirits.

I can dare to dream my wildest dream of who I truly want to be and believe that I become that person. And that this biochemical plant that I call a body can be prepared, through running, stretching, playing, good nutrition, visualization, to receive and enjoy the beauty of my fellow human beings, of the great pictorial and musical works of art, of the fantastic world of nature that is just outside my door. Forty more years of limitless energy, beauty, creativity. Mine to reach out and take.

Training My Transpersonal Will: The Pier

The experience above is an example of how the transpersonal will can be ignited. During the summer of 1977, I used a five-hour swim, performed on the eighth day of a fast, as a means of training my will to overcome negative eating habits and to detoxify my body of aluminum poisoning. The experience was also rich in exercises for training the *transpersonal will* in the face of adversity from within and without.

At the time of the experience, I was living in a lovely rented home in Santa Barabara with my assistant, Vinita Bellandi.

It was a month ago when I first walked down to the beach after having returned from several trips to the East Coast, feeling overfed, under-trained, and generally very polluted.

As I rubbed the oil on my skin I dreamed of some day seeing once again tanned, silken-toned flesh that could excite my inner sense of beauty. Looking out over the water, in the far distance I could see two piers about five miles apart, one on the right, one on the left. The one on the right seemed closer, perhaps a mile and a half away. The one on the left had a white stripe across it. I decided then and there that that would be my trail and that some day I would swim from one pier to the other and back.

Day after day I went into the water and became able to withstand the cold, the fog, the winds, for longer and longer periods of times. During this time, I was working on this book and I wanted my mind clear. I want-ed to be able to articulate my life's work and vision, to inspire others to their health and beauty. So I decided to begin an eight-day juice fast.

The first day I slept and recuperated the full day, staying in bed to read a book by Esther Harding about woman and her mysteries. At that moment I connected to the moon spirit, the fertility rite of the endless powers of the Universe personified in the powers of the moon.

Vinita amd I cooked the vegetables, drank the potassium broth, downed the bran and the flaxseed, and had our carrot juice and other sundry fruit juices. As usual I had my minor slips but this time they were relatively insignificant.

Each day the fast became a living reality. It was almost like living with the twin shadow of my own conciousness as I felt pound after pound slip-ping away. The form of my body started taking shape, the white skin be-coming rich and colored with the rays of the sun and the salt water pene-trating and detoxifying the inner layers of my cellular system. And each day the one-and-a-half-mile swim to the pier on the right seemed to get shorter and shorter. Finally, on the third day, I managed to swim the en-tire way through the seaweed, past the oil spill, to the pier.

The Sixth Day of the Fast

The following day, the sixth day of the fast, I was lying on the beach with Vinita and I gazed to my left at the pier with the white stripe. Casually I commented: "Today I'm going to swim to the furthest pier." And once again I stepped into the water. Stroke after stroke after stroke . . . I felt I was swimming to the beat of an infinite metronome. It seemed endless getting to the pier and I realized it was, indeed, over a two-and-a-half-hour swim. When I had almost gotten to the pier on the left with the white stripe, three and a half miles away, three girls on a rubber raft looked unbelieving at me and said, "We saw you swimming all the way down the coastline. Was that really you?" I was too fatigued to give much of an answer. I went to the pier, touched it almost undramatically, walked into the shore past all the sunbathers and the gorgeous blond, tanned bodies. I met Vinita when I had almost reached our blanket. She and I ran about a quarter of a mile together. I was totally, utterly exhausted.

The following day I stayed home and wrote letters all day. A heavy thick fog set over the city and it was like being in the middle of a tropical rain forest.

The Eighth Day

There's an uncanny clarity that begins to consume your consciousness about the eighth day of the fast. All the senses are heightened. A light begins to grow in your heart and an inner wisdom begins to take over from trivial mundane reality. This quiet sense led Vinita and me to take two cars to the beach today, for I knew that this was the day the pier and I would become one.

Beginning the Ten-mile Swim

Then came the day when I made my first attempt to swim the entire five miles between the two piers.

The water was warm today, very warm. 65 degrees. It was still and I looked out past the Santa Barbara recreation center. The coldness hurt my sunburned skin and as usual I dove in under the water and made a loud yell.

So I started down the coastline, my mind running an endless chatter of nonsensical mutterings. I couldn't get into the swim at all. My arms were heavy, my back was tight. The seaweed, the endless, bobbing seaweed, kept scratching and cutting my sunburned skin. Yet I knew this would be a magical swim.

And all of a sudden I found I was getting into "that space"; that calm, reverie space of personal transcendence. I closed my eyes in the water and I began to dream about establishing a training center here in Santa Barbara. I began to think about my life and the kind of daily training ritual I wanted, of running the mountain every day and coming back to yoga and music and inspiration.

And it was astounding. I began to get into that lilting, rolling flow, watching my left arm sculpt and carve the water gracefully and elegantly as my knees relaxed. And, stroke after stroke, I found myself swimming in the spirit of a Mozart sonata lightly through the warm upper layers of the water. At times I would open my eyes to the murky depth and occasionally gaze down at "the pier." But the distance began to shrink as my consciousness sensed the familiarity of my journey. I sent out an imagined energy streamer and hooked it around the barnacles as I started to visualize the body and the consciousness and the energy I desired. My mind was darting from thought to thought, as a miraculous stream of conciousness flooded me with a kaleidoscopic flow of fleeting impressions of calm serenity.

About a quarter of a mile from the pier, I was suddenly aware, as I looked way, way back, of how far I had come and how easy the swim had been. And how it had been less than a month since I dreamed that by the end of the summer I would be able to swim to the pier. I went past the area where the boats are docked. A slight oil spill lay over the water. I would not allow the negativity to get in the way of my consciousness of swimming to the pier.

Within a few hundred yards I looked up, appreciating the power in my body, and I touched the pillars and came to shore. I had made it, the complete five miles from one pier to the other. I felt strong and light and somehow cleansed.

Halfway There

I went up on the sand for a few minutes, lay down on my back for less than three, and went back into the water to wash off the sand. All of a sudden I made a decision.

"Dyveke, you're going to now swim back, another five miles." My arms and back felt sore. I was a little cold. The oil had gone down. It was about 20 minutes of five. Looking down to the other pier, the distance seemed endless, an almost insurmountable task.

As I waded out into the water, I took a few strokes and was very dismayed. My heart wasn't in it. I thought about getting out again and running down the beach. But I didn't feel like it.

I said, "Dyveke, today you have a unique chance to train your consciousness. Your body is ready to make the swim. DO IT!" So I started.

About three minutes into the swim, I dedicated it to the pier, to Percy Cerutty. I said to myself, "Percy, dear, this swim is for you." And I repeated the phrase he used so often, "Believe in yourself, trust yourself, and never, never quit."

All of sudden my whole attitude changed. The sparkling 80-year-old eyes came into my soul and I thought how I would be at the age of 80, inspiring people to health and beauty and inner wisdom. And I started down the coastline. Within a hundred yards of the pier, I began to look up at the mountains and the palm trees and think how utterly beautiful this area is. I thought how glorious it was that I could swim and have such beauty surrounding me. Memories of the cold, frozen lake in Canada where I swam last summer danced before me and I remembered the logs banging about my head. I found my thoughts elevated by ideas such as "Be true to your own highest convictions."

The water was silken and warm on the surface, and I would stop every now and then to do a backward cartwheel. The bottom layers would be frozen and my legs would cramp, but coming to the surface I could release the cramp immediately.

A beautiful inner joy began to surround me. There was so little seaweed, I could get into the meditative rhythm which allows all the magical spaces to happen.

The Sting

All of a sudden I raised my left hand to put it down in the water and a paralyzing sting coursed through my body. I reared back, thrashed about in the water, and was stunned. My legs and toes cramped. What happened? Fear coursed through me: sharks, jellyfish, sting rays!

"Good God, I am an alien in a hostile environment."

I was shocked out of my reverie. I looked around and could see absolutely nothing. So slowly I made my way to shore, doing a side stroke, unable to use my left arm. I was trying to hold it up and look around. I couldn't see anything on my skin. But I was frightened, terrified for a few minutes.

As I got to shore, my left arm dangling helplessly, I held it up to a young bather throwing a frisbee. He couldn't see anything. He said, "Well, Ma'am, there's been some jellyfish out there, but I haven't seen too many today." I looked out around the ocean. The recreation center seemed far, far away and here I was with a left arm that stung and hurt and was a little paralyzed. I had earlier made a vow to myself. If I could swim back the full length from the pier, I would remain on the fast during the five to six days I would be in Columbus, Ohio. I would do it as a tribute to Vinita and my own personal health. Something in me wanted to keep that promise.

I knew if I got out of the water and lay in the sand my fear would overcome me and I wouldn't go back into the ocean. And I couldn't keep my promise to myself, the fast, Vinita, or Percy. So after I spoke with the young man I realized that the tentacles of a jellyfish had probably splashed against me.

Once more I turned the negative into the positive.

"Dear Beautiful, Living Things of the Ocean, please forgive my intrusion into your territory. I mean you no harm and I know you mean me no harm. Yet I am human and my flesh is soft, so please, Dear Universe, protect me in my swim and guide me."

The feeling began to return to my left arm, and I resumed my slow, gliding strokes.

The water was warm and the distance began to shrink now as, stroke after stroke, I resumed my slow, meditative swim. I found that each time my hands struck a bed of seaweed I jumped. Visions of putting my hand smack into those poisonous jellyfish tentacles danced before me. And my whole body grew taut and frozen as images appeared of a shark rearing up and grabbing me in my belly and tossing me in a pool of blood.

Once again I continued my strokes past the rounded AA building, past the palm trees, past the little flags of the Santa Barbara Inn. And two and a half hours later I had completed the swim back to the pier; a total of ten miles in five hours on the eighth day of a fast.

Aftermath

What a marvelous reward it was to have a strawberry-lemon juice at the health bar l5 minutes later. I looked like a wreck, with my vaseline-soaked hair and red eyes. Externally I was a dirty, sandy fright in a terry cloth robe. Internally I felt like a beauteous Grecian maiden.

That evening, Vinita and I went to the planetarium at the Natural History Museum for an hour-long lecture/demonstration on the Milky Way. Our heads resting on the plush leather cushions, we gazed at galaxies and stars hundreds and thousands and millions of light years away. Before the sheer immensity of the implications of the mystery of the life force, I felt personally dwarfed. Yet my feelings of reverence and awe were amplified by my experiences on the swim.

I thought, "How trivial and mundane our egocentric worlds are when we are less than a mere 'piece of dust' in the universe."

Today, I had experienced something very personal, very transcendent as I trained my body, mind, and spirit to be a larger and more open channel for the incredible universal force that is flowing through me.

Inspiring and Disciplining

As a Coach I want you to see lifestyle training not only as getting your body in shape so that you feel better and doing it in a way that is fun (the left end of the training spectrum), but also to see your training as a time to be working at the other end of the spectrum; the end where you will have moments of tremendous revelation and illumination; where you will overcome negative self-programming and be constantly visualizing that which you want to become. The resulting moments of ecstasy and transcendence will have an incredibly integrating effect on your psyche. They put everything in proper perspective and focus. They can also at times shatter your well-constructed lifestyle.

As a concert artist I have spent years working on a piece, reworking phrases. You too will practice and practice until that day when the most ecstatic electricity goes through you and you have one of those illumined breakthroughs of total transcendence. All of a sudden, all those years of work are validated. You have experienced the upper limit of self-awareness.

So your physical training should be approached with the goal of purposely evoking moments of personal transcendence. I have given examples in this chapter of my own experiences. I've tried to show you how to provoke and stimulate this state in your external environment and your internal mental set.

Men with strong wills have difficulty thinking about the whole matter of the will. Their wills are so strong they can't believe that other people have trouble willing to do something. I know executives who have strong wills, but wills that are one-pointed. They are only directed toward reaching business goals. I have see such men get ignited, begin to train their transpersonal will, and actually turn their lives around as well as the lives of untold others.

Everyone who has tried to do any physical training knows that the whole problem is one of motivation. Self-discipline is seen as applying will power. My message is that we don't usually do what we do just because it is good for us. We do what we enjoy doing and we enjoy doing it because it is fun, inspiring, and joyous. This is what your training time should be. If it isn't, you aren't training correctly and the chances that you will drop out of training are very high. That doesn't mean you will always feel like training when you are scheduled to do so. It doesn't mean you are going to go out and have an ecstatic experience every day. But in the main, your training should be an inspiring and joyful experience.

We must work every single day on inspiring and disciplining the things that we want to believe about ourselves and that we want to see happen in our lives. And we've got to do homework on ourselves to implement those things. This means disciplining and training the will. This is the key to being able to sustain the training program that will be described in the following chapters.

Chapter Four:
Moving the Body

The next step in your Lifestyle Training Program is to start moving. Your moving doesn't have to be running or jogging. It could be walking to work twice a week, getting your bicycle out of the basement and riding for several miles several times a week, investing in and using cross country skis when the winter snows come, resuming your membership at the Y and swimming once or twice a week. The type of moving is not nearly as important as the fact of moving. The essential point is that there is a natural wisdom in the body that kinesthetically comes through when the body is in motion. We are meant to move. Movement is the natural language of the body. And if you do it in the right way, it will become a natural addiction.

From Wheels and Ropes to Tennis Courts

The particular form that your moving takes will depend on your own preferences. The following are examples some of my students have chosen.

Running

One executive uses running as his form of moving. He runs three miles to work at 6:30 in the morning, works for four hours, and then does a brisk two miles at a slightly faster, eight-minute mile, pace. He then has a breakfast of cereals, yogurt, toast, and milk. He had to solve several very fundamental problems in his program of moving. First, he had to work out a way of not getting chilled while he was working after his run. Second, he lives in an area of the country where there is little grass to run on in the winter, so he had to learn to train on busy suburban streets. Third, he had to learn

63

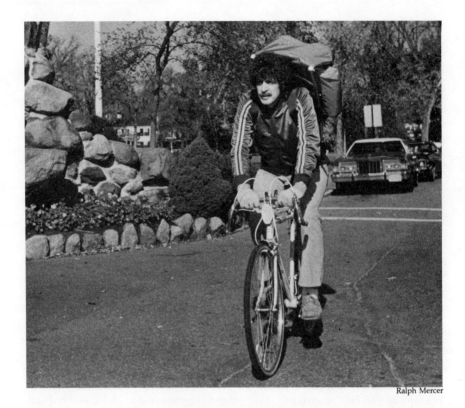

Ralph Mercer

to take care of his feet. He had to discard a favorite old pair of shoes that were causing his toenails to buckle, making blisters on his feet, and pulling his body being out of alignment.

Dotty's training program started with sporadic running and has gradually moved to the point where she is like a beautiful barefoot Indian running over the mountains of Mount Tamalpais. Through her training she overcame her smoking habit and negative self-programming. She also had to overcome her fear of closed areas. I helped her with this by symbolically giving her a Christmas Eve gift of the mountain. I gave her a little branch with a ribbon around it as a way of playfully extending the trail that she would run on. By overcoming her phobia, she made this beautiful mountain her friend.

Bicycling

One marvelous way of starting to move is to ride a bicycle. Many of you have bicycles that are stored in the garage or basement. If you look at your schedule, you may find many times which you could use your bicycle instead of your car, and combine moving with business or errands. One executive I know did just that. Bill was having a hard time keeping his running program going because of having to work many hours of overtime at his office. He had almost given up on physical training when I suggested that he ride his bicycle to work.

His first reaction was, "I haven't ridden a bike in 20 years and I do a lot of traveling. But on my days in the office I do wear jeans." He tried the seven-mile trip one late summer morning. He noted that it only took a few miles to regain the feel of handling the bicycle. He also found that he hardly perspired at all. And, much to his surprise, it took him only about 15 minutes longer to get to work on his bike than to drive, 35 minutes as compared to 20. He immediately began to feel better, more like he felt when he ran regularly. Now, whenever he needs to go to the grocery or hardware store, he goes straight for his bicycle. Bill found that there is more than one way to keep the moving portion of a training program going.

Swimming

I coached one woman in a swimming pool. She began her training program by simply going to a friend's pool and getting in the water twice a week. She didn't even swim. She just went through the motions of putting on a bathing cap and a suit, getting in the water, and taking a sauna afterwards. By activating her sweat glands she created a desire to increase the number of times she went to the sauna. A swimming program evolved naturally.

One famous bioenergeticist who had been a world-class shot putter approached me to awaken the *feminine principle* in his psyche. We started his training program in a small pool, combining the movement of swimming with visualizations. During a run on Mount Tamalpais, I had one of my psychic flashes. I saw a violin string in water and I suddenly realized that the only way this brilliant man could move to the next level of expressing his theoretical ideas required that he awaken the symbolic representation of the violin string: the fragile, artistic, feminine side of himself.

Other people saw him as a bull: hard-headed, driving, aggressive. I experienced him completely differently. One of the breakthroughs of his training and our relationship occurred when we were able to touch that aspect of his personality long hidden from the public. While swimming, he visualized that beautiful, delicate violin string, and as the music was going through his body it was as though that string was being plucked. All this occurred in a pool while he wore a snorkel and used mental imagery as I walked back and forth "sending him energy."

Tennis

With Jerry, a psychiatrist, the movement in his training program came on the tennis court. When he started his training he was working 14 hours a day, saw patients every 50 minutes, healed children by hypnosis and auto-suggestion, and ran a healing center. He drove himself into the ground and developed hypertension. All this spilled over into his tennis game. I began to help him implement the techniques he teaches everybody else all day but somehow has had difficulty putting into effect in his own life: deep relaxation, getting in touch with feelings, taking time for himself.

My entire coaching of Jerry was simply to reflect back to him his own techniques, and I did this through visualizations. I had him imagine he was throwing up a light streamer into the air, that he was hitting the tennis ball as though it were a wisp of air, that he was spinning his hips as though they were soft pools of water. And I had him apply all the techniques of visualization, meditation, and deep relaxation to the game of tennis. Then I designed a spinal flexibility exercise to balance out the rigidity in his body caused by years of abuse and overwork. Jerry already had the movement going, but it was out of sync with the rest of his life.

Rope Climbing

I coached one very busy engineer who worked all night. His entire training program consisted of going up and down four floors of a sewage treatment plant on a rope that hung outside his window. It wasn't long before we expanded his program include swimming four to five times a week.

There is a natural, instinctive wisdom in the body that can be tapped once we start moving. And what you must do in your training is to plug into that natural instinct playfully, joyously, and with inner awareness. It may be through running, swimming, tennis, or even walking. But the important thing is to start moving and plug in.

From Par-Course to Vita-Course

It was a delight to wind my way through a park in Arlington, Massachusetts, and see a sign proclaiming, "Vita Course" emerging from the fall-colored trees. Developed in Switzerland, the Vita Course has a walking or running trail and a series of openings with pieces of outdoor equipment to fully exercise the body. The first stop, about 100 yards into the trail, called for toe-touching exercises with ten repetitions. Next, upper torso swings. The third, fourth, and fifth stations included hanging bars, swinging rings, and graduated bars to do sit-ups. I especially liked being able to hang upside down, feel the rush of blood to my head, and see the world from bottom up. I noticed my back and legs were stretched in a new way. The combination of the running, scenery, playful equipment, and the obvious workout to hidden muscle sets was exhilarating.

In San Francisco, at the Marina Green, a Par Course has been set up along a newly installed running track. There are 26 stations and each one works the body in a slightly different way, for example, doing sit-ups or stepping up and down log stumps. This particular course winds around grassy fields, out along a beach, with a path to an old fort underneath the Golden Gate Bridge. One's training time is filled with vistas, ocean breezes, and the pleasure, of sharing your workout with others.

I personally believe these courses will greatly enhance the overall fitness level of the American public as they catch on along with tennis and running. For one thing, they tend to *build community*. People go to meet their friends and share a common cause, training in a way that makes it fun. If there is a Par Course or Vita Course in your neighborhood, I heartily recommend that you incorporate it into your schedule. If one is not available, there may be sponsors who will build one. A colleague of mine and former running student, Tom Purvis, who now has a high position in the Public Health Department, enticed the city to install a Par Course at a nearby park because of his interest in running and fitness.

Aikido

Aikido is one of the highest forms of sport in which we can participate. As a form of exercise it is outstanding. Not only does it afford sufficient cardiovascular training, but also flexibility and concentration. More importantly, the nature of the sport teaches you *how to live in the New Age* by connecting and interchanging energy with another from a place of centered, devotional oneness. In Aikido, one touches and moves with a dancelike grace, developing qualities of character that emulate an evolution of consciousness from one of combat and aggressiveness to focus, decisiveness, and action with flowing harmony.

George Leonard, author of *The Ultimate Athlete*, first introduced me to this beautiful sport. He turned his dining room into an Aikido Dojo. In place of a table and chairs, he had a mat. Two years later, his studio in Mill Valley has become the focal point of many classes and an expanding community of athletes. Most students of Aikido take a monthly membership and train at least three times a week, for one to three hours. It tends to assume a preeminent place in a person's life. Many students train daily. The only disadvantage is the time element and need for a space and other people. Aikido builds unity both within oneself and with others and affords a marvelous way to find companionship while embarking on a Lifestyle Training Program.

Indoor Equipment

One of the most useful pieces of indoor equipment is a mini-trampoline. These can be used for a full workout, instant energizing, and play. Dr. Norman Shealey, Director of the Pain Clinic in La Crosse, Wisconsin, uses a trampoline in the corner of his bedroom each morning for 20 minutes. Lifting his legs high and prancing, he avoids the cold weather and works up a good sweat. My friend, Chuck, plays music and frolics while his pulse shoots up to 200. I recommend this for anyone anticipating a running program, for it can provide training for those with tight schedules and tone and tighten long unused muscles before a full-fledged training program is started. A good small trampoline costs between $125 - $175.

A slant board is excellent for sit-ups and leg raises and combined with a jump rope can afford an excellent training program. There are many commercial gadgets around to facilitate *moving*. It is unnecessary here to go into detail regarding pros and cons. I am concentrating on what you can do *on your own* without investing in expensive equipment. A stationary exercise bicycle, mini-trampoline, and jump rope are the three best tools for indoor cardiovascular exercise.

Ball Sports

Part of training for many people is to get in shape so that they can play ball sports such as basketball, racketball, squash, football, rugby. . . . The purpose of this book is to help you learn to *play and stay in good health all your life*, and, I hope, with a different attitude toward competition. It is extremely difficult for most of us to embark on a Lifestyle Training Program by playing a ball sport. It takes too much time, and the twisting, jerking, leaping, and banging activates old injuries and puts undue strain on underworked muscles. We want to get in shape to play our sport, not use our sport to try to get in shape.

One of the reasons I became a New Age Coach was because of the terrible abuses I saw in the bodies and minds of people attempting sports they were not in condition to play. At Squaw Valley, it broke my heart to see so many twisted and broken legs and ankles. I started a series of classes in pre-season ski conditioning to introduce the techniques of proper endurance, strength, flexibility, sensing, and innerspace. This included "how to read the mountain by intuition, as to snow, wind, and skiing conditions."

And the same is true with tennis. The shock and pounding the spine and joints take is enormous. It is devastating to an unused body. For five years I taught Tennis Flow at Esalen Sports Center to help people train properly with running, weights, stretching, and visualization to control the powers of the mind before hitting hundreds of tennis balls on a concrete court.

All ball sports are exhilarating and should be joyous. But first you must lay the base.

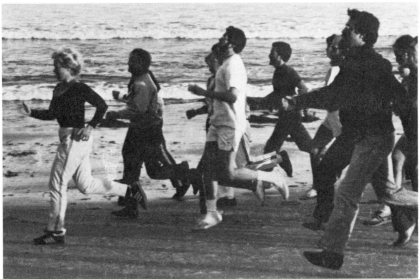

Sandy Solomon

Moving Is Important

The main reason for moving is not to lose weight or to look more attractive, but to develop a more efficient system for delivering oxygen to the cells. A consequence of a more efficient delivery system is that you feel more energetic, and the quality of your energy is higher. Because you are carrying fewer toxins in your cellular system, you tend to need less sleep, and the whole accumulation of cultural stress is diminished.

There are certain principles that you need to know about how your bodily functions. First, you are an ambulatory mammal moving in relation to gravity. In your movement you are propelling blood throughout your body. Your endurance, your body's ability to handle stress loads, is based on the capacity of your most important muscle, the heart, to facilitate the flow of blood. The reason for endurance or aerobic training is to extend your network of capillary endings. This is the essence of increasing the body's ability to utilize oxygen through the flow of blood to the heart and increasing the capillary supply of that blood flow throughout the body.

About the Heart

The heart is a demand pump: it will pump as hard and as often as the demand is made on it. Exercise presents the heart with a demand. If you present this demand in a controlled fashion with gradual build-up, the heart will learn to respond so that when you climb a mountain, run up a flight of stairs, shovel snow, or introduce some other stress, the heart is prepared. If it is not, you could be in serious trouble.

The heart responds to demand by pumping harder and faster, in the same fashion that a bicep responds to the demand of a dumb-bell that is being lifted. And the same thing happens to the heart that happens to the bicep. It grows. It becomes bigger and stronger. Any of the moving exercises — swimming, running, bicycling, jumping rope, running up the stairs — puts a demand on the heart that can help to increase its efficiency.

No one with any history of heart, pulmonary, or kidney disease should attempt to start any cardiovascular or aerobic program without first a having a really good physical examination and a complete discussion of the program with his or her doctor. Putting a demand on the heart from an exercise like running, delivers as much as 70% of the blood to the muscles of the legs, the upper torso, and the peripheral skin. Thus the kidneys, liver, and all the other internal organs are going to be short-changed. If you start out with heart or kidney problems, you may be asking for trouble.

Blood Pressure and Hypertension

High blood pressure is the number one killer and is related to hypertension. It becomes doubly evident why I am encouraging people to train with a joyous attitude and a loving feeling state: we simply don't need to add more tension to an already hyper-tense society. We need to alter our consciousness about the way we conduct our lives and the things we value.

As pointed out in a recent article by James Hassett, associate editor of *Psychology Today* (Pg. 31-40, August, 1978):

> The hardest and most important muscle in the body beats an average of 70 times per minute, 100,000 times each day or more than 2 ½ billion times in 70 years. It pumps about 1800 gallons of blood each day. In a lifetime, that totals 46 billion gallons. The force required to pump this much blood, if it could be harnessed in a single instant, would lift a ten ton weight 10 miles in the air. In the body, this force circulates the blood through an incredible labyrinth of blood vessels that if laid end to end would stretch from Boston to Hoboken, New Jersey, and back more than 150 times; something on the order of 62,000 miles.

> Blood pressure is the force of the blood moving away from the heart pushing against the artery walls. It changes from instant to instant, peaking as the heart beats and blood spurts through the arteries and gradually decreases to a minimum just before the next beat. Blood pressure is expressed in two numbers, the systolic pressure, the maximum valve, when the heart beats *over* the diastolic pressure, the minimum pressure between beats. It is measured in millimeters of mercury.

> More Americans die of cardiovascular problems than all other causes of death combined. Only half of the 46 million Americans with high blood pressure are even aware of their problems. Life insurance companies say that blood pressure is the single best predictor of how long a person

will live. A 35-year-old man with a blood pressure of 150/100 for instance will probably die 16 years earlier than one with normal pressure of 120/80.

Biofeedback can reduce blood pressure but studies show that its effects don't always last after the subject leaves the lab. Teaching a person to relax is harder than prescribing pills. And doctors lack the training and inclination.

As stated earlier, my personal belief is that frightening statistics may be one, but not primarily the most powerful, *ignition switch* to get people to move. It is my experience that igniting the will through beauty, inspiration, and joy, and exciting and motivating the *transpersonal will* is far more long-lasting.

Hypertension is a direct result of competition, garbage food, and lack of exercise, as well as being out of touch with our feelings and nature. As Dr. Stephen Bajon, pharmacist turned nutritionist who recovered from diabetes, said: "I want to help bring *peace* on this planet. To my mind, the reason we've never had peace on this planet is because people have not been properly nourished. How can we be relaxed and in a non-stress state if we are not properly nourished? Nourishment brings peace. There are a lot of jangled people running around because their biochemistry is out of balance. Hypertension is the direct result of improper nutrition, not moving or not being in touch with our spiritual nature."

Long Distance Endurance Training

In the moving portion of my Lifestyle Training Programs, I subscribe to the methods of long slow distance endurance training which are in harmony with all the other principles of body flow and structural alignment of the skeletal muscle frame. They are conducive to deep states of mental relaxation and are the most natural to our ambulatory nature, which is to cover distance, playfully and joyously, without undue pain or strain. These methods are also most conducive to awakening the *feminine principle* since competition is minimized and motivation comes from an *inner sense of being in touch with feelings*.

Van Aaken on Endurance Training

In an article entitled "The Endurance Function in Theory and Practice," translated by George Beinhorn, Dr. Ernst Van Aaken succinctly describes long distance slow training:

Endurance training consists predominantly of long distance training at a slow pace, daily in any weather, in forest, on streets and roads, with many walking pauses and very occasional sprint runs. Total recovery is sought during the walking pauses. Endurance training strives to create an increase in aerobic metabolism by keeping stresses constantly at the

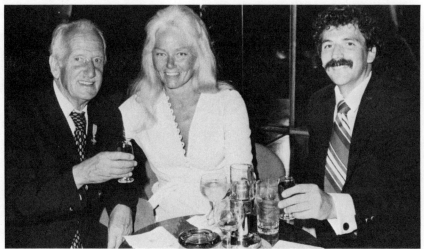

From left to right: Mike Spino, Dyveke Spino, Percy Wells Cerutty.

point of optimal breathing efficiency, i.e., the maximum absorption of oxygen from the smallest volume of air. This occurs at a pulse rate between 120 and 140. If at all possible, avoid anaerobic functioning and formation of lactic acid. In endurance training an increase in the heart's volume is created by continuous low-intensity stresses over a long period of time, two to six years.

Van Aaken also says in an article entitled "The Training of the Future":

A runner who is best provided with oxygen, because of his oxygen training — endurance training at a slow pace — will always storm off faster in the long dash over the last laps, because he still has oxygen reserves and is thus completely fresh . . . the most important principal is that *one learns to run by running*.

Pritikin and Roving

Van Aaken's approach is essentially the same as the famed Pritikin method of physical fitness as outlined in the book: *Live Longer Now*. Pritikin suggests *roving*, which is a system of measuring off a distance and systematically walking and running it four to five times a week to build up endurance. Pritikin stresses that the runner not pay attention to time but to distance with the purpose being to "satisfy your urge to run." I was immensely impressed with the simple, natural wisdom of this physical training program, for its purpose is not to compete with yourself or others but just *go out there and do it*. And I saw the results last summer in Santa Barbara where clients at his center jogged, walked, danced, stretched, and swam up and down the same coastline where I swam every day, and did it with an attitude of fun and playfulness.

Percy Cerutty and Naturalistic Running

Why is it that one learns to run by running? Is it because an instinctive wisdom begins to surface in our consciousness about survival? It was on the *instinct towards survival* that Percy Wells Cerutty based his entire training system: live with the natural elements, eat uncooked food, stay close to beauty and your feelings, and dare to have the courage to believe in yourself. All of this must be based upon having a fit, strong body in touch with the *will to survive*.

Cerutty's training system was based on naturalistic rhythms and gaits that emulated the patterns of animals, especially horses, moving. His methods of endurance training, which produced many world class athletes in all sports as well as Olympic record-holders, taught people how to run barefoot in the woods for long distances, to play with the natural elements, to sleep in Spartan surroundings (sometimes in very cold temperatures), and to run like a horse: gallop, trot, canter, ambulate freely over the ground with loose shoulders and wrists. Cerutty wrote nine books published by Putnam Press of England. They are out of print but still available through some libraries.

Cerutty resurrected his own health after being seriously ill by taking long hikes with a pack on his back and gradually starting to run. He lived to be 80 and continued to break Australian records and train world class athletes and others interested in reclaiming their health.

Cerutty believed that most athletes did not realize their potential because they did not properly fill their lungs with oxygen. He developed a technique called *full lung aeration* in which lifting the arms, taking in air, exhaling and making noises, can bring more oxygen into the lungs. This requires five basic arm movements.

Cerutty was also a staunch believer in weight training. His system used heavy weights with few repetitions to build inner-tensile muscle power without bulk. The five lifts are: (1) one-arm swing, (2) cheat curl, (3) bench press, (4) dead lift and (5) sit-ups. The athlete lifted the heaviest possible weight with only five repetitions per set with a limit of two or three sets. Weight training was alternated with gynmastics workouts on ropes, bars, vaults, and trampoline to develop balance and coordination. This was combined with sand-hill running.

I believe Percy Cerutty was one of the greatest coaches of all time, not only because he *returned to nature* to develop his beliefs and system, but because he instinctively knew the *power of the will* and importance of training it systematically with inspiration. (This will be discussed in the following chapter.) Cerutty also understood the relationship of each aspect of training to the whole, for instance, the vitality that comes from eating organic food, freshly picked.

He also realized the importance of retraining the neurological patterns of the brain which are *grooved* by set and rote patterns of movement. He believed these movements, such as locked elbows, caused rigidity in one's sponteneity and ability to express movement rhythmically in a flowing way similar to animals. Cerutty's ideas resemble those of Dr. Moshe Feldenkrais who developed a remarkable system of exercises to *increase the range of motion* throughout the body by retraining the neurological patterns of the brain using slow, meditative exercises done in a state of non-resistance to gravity. (This is discussed in Chapter 7 on Flexibility.)

In 1973, the Esalen Sports Center brought Percy Cerutty to the United States and he lived with me and my former husband, Mike Spino, while conducting a series of clinics and workshops to teach his methods of naturalistic movement. Despite Cerutty's sometimes difficult behavior, he was a great inspiration to me. His close friend Bill Emmerton accompanied us on part of this tour. Bill, one of the world's greatest ultra-long distance runners, described training sessions with Cerutty in Australia in which the two would copy the movements of gazelles, antelopes, and the aborigines.

Cerutty's body at the age of 80 was light, fluid, strong, and his skin was silken. I connected with Cerutty at an artistic and emotional level. He confided, "I never meant to be a coach. I just had to learn to survive for myself and the lads started coming to me. I wanted to go to Paris and study art but I was too sickly and poor." Indeed, Cerutty's great gift was his ability to ignite and inspire the impossible. His saying: "believe in yourself, trust yourself, and never, never quit" is one that I find myself repeating over and over to my students.

I now teach Cerutty's training methods, the various rhythms and gaits, and can attest to the joy and fluidity that beginning and advanced runners experience. This expression through movement fosters emotional sponteneity with the end result that training is more interesting and fun. I am the only woman in the world Cerutty certified to teach his training methods.

Starting to Move

My job as a New Age Coach is to help you get the moving process started. It's very simple: if you love yourself, you just have to start *moving*. Once you have decided to start moving, you will have to decide how. How you start to move will depend on your schedule and your lifestyle, including the things you want for yourself: your goals, your aspirations, your dreams. These are all things you examined in Chapter 2. Percy Cerutty began the long process of resurrecting his health by going on long, long walks and hikes. He put a pack on his back as a form of weight training. He did a lot of his walking and hiking up and down hills which put an extra stress load on his body.

Once you start moving in accordance with the principle of long, slow distance training, the payoff is so immediate you will realize that it is a self-propelling system of positive addiction of the type Glasser talks about in his book *Positive Addiction*. The process is truly like a drop of water that starts to melt ice. It will eventually pervade every aspect of your life.

If you decide that your moving is to be running, the way to begin is to combine walking and running for a certain distance or for a certain period of time. Your body will give you clues as to which. Just be sure to do it regularly. Percy Cerutty agreed with this approach. You simply take 30 to 40 minutes per day for three to four days a week and walk a little bit and run a little bit. Don't carry a stop watch or pay undue attention to how far you've gone. Simply go out for a period of time, or designate a distance that is reasonable for your level of fitness and your time demands. You will find that after a few times you will start to extend your running time almost automatically.

My personal preference for a training program is a combination running/swimming program. It would begin with running three times a week and swimming at least once a week. Because swimming is non-weight bearing, it stretches out the skeletal muscle system and allows the energy flow of the body to become naturally balanced.

As you get into some kind of moving, either walking or walking mixed with gentle jogging, think about places in your environment which you can utilize to put on extra stress loads. I remember when I first started to coach Dr. Stanley Krippner, we designed a training program that involved walking up the hill behind his office, followed by jogging very lightly down a very steep flight of steps and then running on a flat place. Finally, we found a little trail through some eucalyptus trees near his office.

Two months later, as his conditioning got better, he would do his workout at the nearby park. He would run down the street and do more strenuous workouts on the hills in the park, which were very steep. We would playfully run around trees, up and down the hills, sometimes with bystanders clapping their hands or delighting in our fun. And then there were three months when he had a heavy travel schedule of foreign cities and motels. He would sometimes do his training in the hallways of the hotel, on the stairs, or in a nearby grass field. And when it was raining very heavily in Paris, he did a lot of rope jumping.

I've designed programs for women who, housebound by little babies, were buying diet foods loaded with preservatives and food additives in an attempt to lose weight. They would do sit-ups in their living room with their feet tucked under the couch. Their cardiovascular work was simply running up and down the stairs. Their stretching was hanging on the moldings around the house. And a lot of their limbering and flexibility work was done simply by wearing tights and a leotard during the day and caring for the baby.

In the next chapter we are going to talk in detail about the importance of the care of the spine and skeletal muscle flexibility. But you should be aware that everything you do when moving must be interwoven with flexibility work. There are simple, elementary flexibility exercises that you can and should do in conjunction with your moving. For instance, suspend a rope somewhere in your immediate environment and just hang on the rope or go hand over hand.

Slowly and Playfully

It is astounding to me to read the Van Aaken material on edurance training. Van Aaken is a great German scientist, physician and sports training expert, with an excellent scientific training laboratory. He reported that the net result of all his findings was that we were to run long, run slow, run joyously and playfully. Remember that: run long, run slow, run joyously and playfully. As you start to move, make a game out of it. Play with yourself, become a child again. Go and watch children as they run and move and play and swing and jump and twist. That is what we are meant to do our entire lifetime.

In Boston last winter, every time there was a beautiful new fresh snow storm, you would see all the children clambering around on garage roofs having a great time with snowballs. For the adults it was just drudgery. That's what Cerutty always talked about. If you want to learn anything, watch children play, watch how they move. And watch animals.

Forming a Support System

When you start to move, you may feel that you need a strong support group, especially if you're a woman. So your first moving may be in a yoga class three times a week. This could be a good beginning but yoga in and of itself may not be strenuous enough to give you sufficient cardiovascular conditioning.

A lot of men reading this are like Bob, who I am now coaching. Bob does some of his moving with a support group, a rugby team. At the age of 30, he gained a lot of weight. Now he is playing rugby. He started to get his body moving first by a very intensive year-and-a-half progam of weight training. But he realized that the possiblity of injuries in rugby meant that he had to move his body in different ways to help prepare himself for the game. So training for him now means an entire system of detoxification from improper nutrition and improper balances in the endocrine system. This includes body work and altering his running style from hard sprint work to long, slow distance.

So, for you, starting to move may mean that you have to invest the money to join a health club or to take a series of classes. But I also encourage you to do the simplest, most obvious thing which is to change your environment in your own home and working situation by simple things such as ropes and pulleys, a slant board, a little trampoline, a jump rope, a set of weights. And then get on some kind of walking and running program.

How You Will Feel

When they first start to move, most people feel heavy, waterlogged, their insides bounce. Women feel terrible because their breasts hurt and their buttocks and legs feel too big. What you have to realize is that we have not only a sugar-addicted culture, we have a salt-addicted one as well. Intercellular fluids are retained in your skeletal muscle system, because of the sodium addiction in our culture. When you first start to move, you want to get salt totally out of your diet, so you must find a book that gives the sodium content of foods, and you might do as I do and carry a list of low sodium foods. I loved Swiss cheese but it was the highest of all foods in sodium content!

When you first start to train, the heaviness you feel is the result of being waterlogged. Consequently, when you first start to move you will sweat a lot, but as you get in better and better physical condition you won't have that drenching wetness all the time. A woman who is starting to move needs a good bra. And don't worry about feeling so flabby and soft. We all are unless we really move our bodies. With men it is very much the opposite. They feel a great deal of tightness in their legs and their upper shoulders, the accumulated stress of the competitive culture, so they feel really heavy when they start to move their bodies.

When you move, you have to get through that first phase which feels foreign and uncomfortable and unnatural. This is where the attitude of playfulness can be very important.

Creative Running

There's more to running than putting one foot in front of the other with some degree of speed and rhythm. There is also the possibility of transforming your consciousness to transcend physical limitations, to reach toward magical spaces of ecstasy and oneness with the universe, toward structural harmony and internal flow.

When you first start to run, be very gentle and kind to yourself. Let the feminine side of yourself nurture and protect and care for you. Be sensitive to feelings. Most people don't train this way. They tear up to a track in their cars, jam on the brakes, jump out, and take off at full tilt around the track. This is the yang energy, the masculine energy. They want to get there and work as fast and as hard as they can. They get shin splints, pulled Achilles tendons, and all kinds of injuries, because they don't realize what they are doing. They don't integrate running with the rest of their lives. How often I feel a quiet pain when I watch crumpled runners banging on pavement, taking in lead poisoning, thinking they are getting *fit* when just a few hundred yards away is a beautiful grass field where they could undulate their spines, take in the prana of the grass, and fill their lungs with fresh oxygen.

Preparation for Running

The best time to run is around dawn, just as the sun is rising, when the prana is at the apex, the air cleaner, and your mind uncluttered by the demands of the day. Ideally, you should run in a beautiful place, on soft grass, through the woods, or around a lake or reservoir. Be especially careful to avoid getting chilled. It's best to wear loose cotton (rather than synthetic) clothing and to dress on the warm rather than the cool side. Especially at the beginning, wear long pants to keep the muscles warm. And pay attention to the obvious. Don't stop to chat with a friend when you've worked up a big sweat. Elevate your training to a feeling of becoming an artist with your body. Treat it with extreme care and delicacy. Wear good running shoes: nylon is preferable to leather because nylon shoes hold their shape and don't retain water.

Setting the Mood

Setting the mood and tone of your feeling state before training takes only a few minutes and can evoke the heroic and transcendent in you. (See the Meditation for Runners at the end of the chapter.) Maybe you want to arrange your environment so that you wake up to an inspirational scroll with affirmations and desires that you can implant in your consciousness, or to the swell and vibrance of Mozart descending into your cellular system before your run. This may be as important as the run itself. When I get my runners doing this, their whole type-A compulsive driving behavior balances to an inner calm and personal reverence.

Finding a Place to Run

Once you have set the mood for your run, go out and explore your environment. Find a grassy field or a soft dirt track that is flat. I find that most people in the beginning do not pay attention to the most obvious things which are: checking out the grass field near you, taking a look at your environment in another way, finding out where there are soft patches along the road, inspirational areas, little hills you can go up and down.

Before the Run: STRRRRETCH!

Before starting your run, spend at least 15 minutes doing gentle stretching exercises and/or the yoga sun worship series. This set of exercises stretches the spine in seven directions. (See Chapter Seven for other pre-run stretching routines.)

Dictate the following very slowly onto a tape cassette. Then listen and follow the instructions.

1. Lie on your back. Close your eyes and relax deeply. Go inside of your body and sense the holding patterns on the right side and left side of your body. Feel how each foot turns out.
2. Slowly lift both legs over your head and allow your knees to fall beside your ears. Breathe and hold, relaxing into the stretch.
3. Very slowly, uncurl your spine, coming back down on the floor one vertebra at a time.
4. Lift your right leg to a knee-to-chest position, then place it to the right side of your body. Slowly roll the bent right leg across your body and place it on the floor on the opposite (left) side. Extend your right arm straight up above your head, on the floor, and turn your head to the right. Once you are in this position, imagine that there is a golden ball in the center of the earth, spinning rapidly and pulling you deeper and deeper into the earth. Allow your shoulders and knee to sink into the ground. Breathe deeply, then uncurl yourself slowly, coming back to a prone position.
5. Repeat the same stretch on the left side: left leg over the body to the opposite side, left arm up straight over the head. Look to the left. Uncurl back to the prone position.
6. Place both hands behind your neck and slowly curl up to a sit-up position. Hang out over your legs with knees straight. Relax into the stretch, but don't bounce.
7. Very slowly uncurl your spine again, coming down to the floor one vertebra at a time, starting from the small of the back.
8. With bent knees, slowly tilt up the pelvic area and lift up with head and neck remaining on the floor. Slowly come back down, one vertebra at a time, starting from the neck.
9. Close your eyes and once again sense the alignment of your body, left and right. Notice any changes that may have occurred since you began the stretches.
10. Let yourself be in a calm, quiet space, aware of yourself: the inner alignment and feelings of your body. With this quiet awareness, slowly get up and begin your run.

The Run

Start by running slowly, lightly on the feet, going from the heel to the toe, slightly toeing in. Start doing what is called the *shake-up*. Dangle the body from the shoulders, through the hips and ankles. Keep your pace at what is called the nine-minute-mile pace, which is slightly above a fast walk. Work yourself at a pace such that you are breathing hard but are not out of breath or straining anything in your body. Do this for 15 or 20 minutes, three times a week, and in six weeks you will naturally increase your time, distance, and frequency, and will have laid what is called a long, slow distance base. There's no need to constantly push yourself past your limits: just go out and start moving. In order to increase your intake of oxygen, use the "talk test." If you can carry on a conversation as you run, you are in an aerobic state.

You don't have to run in a competitive spirit, either with yourself or with another person. As you run along very slowly, doing the shake-up, the layers of tension and deep holding begin to loosen and reform into more harmonious patterns of "flow." For the experienced athlete or jogger, consciously slowing yourself down for long periods of time is imperative. Sense the alignment of your body, the fluidity of your skeletal muscle frame, the deep relaxation of all the muscle sets, and open your mind to the edges of your own personal ecstasy. The actual incremental time increase to nick off seconds is much less important than overall mental, spiritual, and physical health.

Once you are running, start to play with the recesses and reserves of your inner self. (In the next chapter I will outline specific innerspace exercises you can experiment with.)

Rhythms and Tempos

Eighty percent of your training should be long, slow distance. The other 20 percent should involve rhythms, tempos, percussions, and accelerations. For instance, run backwards, sideways. Jump and twirl. Shout out your ideals or release them as mental pictures in balloons. Do short, fast steps, pumping your arms up and down, focusing your energy on fast step repeats, loudly making the sound of a bee (beeeee!). Feel the explosive and percussive effects of your accelerated energy flow. It's no different from the exultation of experiencing the brilliance of Bach or the harmonies of Bartok. Run with your hands on your hips, lifting your knees high in front of you, feeling the grandeur of a prancing horse.

Lift your shoulders high as you breathe in deeply, and exhale quickly by dropping the shoulders, making a loud guttural noise as the air is released.

Make noise, hear yourself. Touch your primordial, primitive self and allow your unconscious to explode into your body.

Run asymmetrically, galloping or loping like a horse. This tends to extend normal thought patterns, getting you out of the "groove," and bringing creative reintegration.

After any percussive or energetic movements, return to the calm rhythm of the shake-up and recover gracefully and flowingly. The purpose of these techniques is to sensitize and awaken both the male and female energies in the psyche, and to experience them directly and simultaneously.

How to End Your Training

Always end your training with another 15 minutes of stretching, e.g, the yoga triangle pose, forward bends, or hanging over an elevated leg. Don't bounce. Breathe into the stretch, find the edge and relax into it. Steam baths and massage are a good adjunct to physical training, greatly accelerating the elimination of toxins, and encouraging new cell growth. The most important aspect of this type of training program is to learn to get in touch with yourself at all levels. The distance, the pace, the variations, will all evolve naturally and organically once the cardiovascular system becomes exercised and detoxified. The endocrine system starts functioning in balance and both hemispheres of the brain are purring harmoniously. Twenty minutes of running, four to five times a week, plus 20 minutes of flexibility work done in a state of reverence and relaxation, can transform your life.

Rituals

Rituals are a great aid in training your will or directing your intentionality to a repetition of desired behavior. Rituals also reinforce your spirit and help you retain a sense of dedication to your training.

Give a daily greeting to certain trees or beautiful places along your running trail. Circle around a particular tree each day to feel its energy, and treat certain rocks or shrubs as friends welcoming you, on your way. Each day, place a rock at a special place and watch them multiply, a testament to your steady progress. (One such pile helped me run high up on Mount Tamalpais every day.)

Find a beautiful spot along the way to stop and meditate. Find different trees, representing different aspects of yourself, to meditate on. If you run by water, take five minutes to become one with the water. Allow your consciousness to drift into a drop of water and become everlasting life. On my morning runs I often sit on a rock overlooking the ocean and touch the curled bark of a eucalyptus branch. It reminds me of ancient parchment and Gregorian chants. The inspiration of the ritual sometimes inspires me to compose original music.

Creative expression is a natural result of this kind of training and you can finish your ritual off by writing in a journal, or playing the piano or other musical instrument. The fresh oxygen to all cells, the pageantry of nature, the sense of personal integration, may bring forth the dormant artist in you.

In any case, allow yourself to indulge in a "reward" as part of your ritual, be it a special juice you like to drink after running or a special-smelling soap or talcum powder. After all, you deserve it.

The Mind and Physical Training: Therapeutic Effects

For many years, as a psychotherapist and New Age Coach, I was aware of the connection between the therapeutic effects of physical exercise and the ability to reach the subconscious mind. In most of my workshops there are emotional and psychological breakthroughs revealing hidden traumas and buried fears that erupt spontaneously during or following a workout.

My approach is to present myself first as a "coach" and move into the role of psychotherapist when the appropriate circumstance presents itself, e.g., eruption of long-buried fears, phobias, depression, negative self-image beliefs. Some of my consultation sessions are essentially therapy sessions. I try to focus and direct the interchange toward the *positive*. This tends to move the relationship toward one of *colleagueship* rather than *client-patient*.

Recently this field has begun to receive more recognition. An article in *Newsweek*, May 1978, titled "Jogging for the Mind," reports on the work of psychiatrist Thaddeus Kostrubala who practices psychotherapy while jogging with his patients. He believes that jogging makes people more talkative and breaks down the social barrier between therapist and patient. The article states that some doctors prescribe jogging rather than pills for depression. The American Medical Joggers Association, a group of 3,000 jogger-doctors, is starting a program titled "Jungian Talk-and-jog Therapy" at Malibu Beach. A. H. Ismail, Professor of Physical Education at Purdue University, states that running cures some mental problems such as depression by changing the chemical composition of the body. A study has been proposed to the National Institute of Mental Health to test this theory.

I believe this development will result in some of the most creative and potentially useful work in this area. I stumbled into it naturally when I began to feel that working in offices, sitting in chairs, wasn't necessarily the best way to promote human growth. I believe when people are *moving* outside in an inspirational setting, with others, and are exposed to techniques that open up the powers of the mind, the unconscious processes of the mind can't help but release long-buried charges. And as was also noted in the *Newsweek* article: "After 14 to 18 miles of a marathon, people often break

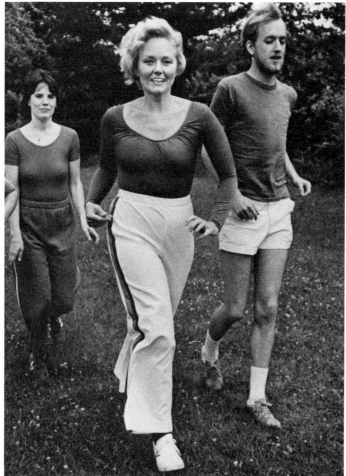

Ralph Mercer

down and cry, or babble to strangers about their childhood memories and problems; exactly the kind of breakthrough that conventional talk therapists look for." This type of breakthough is quite common in my workshops.

Summary: When Moving, Bring Along the Feminine Principle

It is important when you start moving to bring along all the other elements that we have been talking about: that you simultaneously discipline your will and your transpersonal will, that you apply what we have described as the feminine principle, i.e., that you see everything you do as related to everything else. It's no good to increase the oxygen supply to your cells and increase the flow of blood to your heart unless you are also cleaning up improper nutrition. If you are downing cokes, eating hot dogs loaded with red dye and DDT, eating french fries cooked in carcinogenic oil, you will be undoing the benefits of your cardiovascular training.

As you start to move, constantly awaken in yourself the possiblity of tapping into the upper limits. But don't overdo it. This is not what moving the body is about. As my Boston rugby player said, "If I was going slow and feeling good about it, I was feeling guilty that I wasn't hurting enough. And if I was hurting too much, I felt I was satisfying something inside of me, but I wanted to stop." You must find balance.

There are charts and graphs and scientific ways that all this can be measured, but I have found that the single most important thing is igniting the spirit, igniting the inner sense of our own wisdom, like that little seed that has the natural wisdom within it to grow. All of us want to move to the next natural level of our own personal evolution, of our own internal perfection.

Prelude to
Awakening the
Feminine Principle

Exploring Innerspace

During our entire lifetime, we search to be understood. We search for another to gently touch and caress who we are, what we are feeling, our dreams, and to appreciate what we have overcome. This search "to be understood" and "to understand ourselves" requires tapping into the hidden recesses of our subconscious mind, our archetypal self, our "soul"; indefinable, mysterious, seething, as waters that swirl about a tide, coming and going from sculptured rocks.

Our personal history cascades into our consciousness, blending a past, present, and future, perhaps even countless "past lives," into a stream of consciousness, the accumulation of which adds up to the "I" you are experiencing.

This innerspace is virtually uncharted territory, and I am one of the few coaches extensively using it to facilitate "turning within and listening."

One of my students gives this account of innerspace work at a workshop in Toronto:

> We were all anxious to start moving. But Dyveke was saying, "Lie down on the grass on your backs. Put your arms by your side with the palms up and close your eyes. Let your whole body just sink into the grass. Let all the stiffness go. Let your mind be quiet. Let the sounds of the breeze through the trees flow through your body."
>
> It was a perfect day to be outside. The sun was shining brightly from a sky with no clouds. The grass on the rolling hills of the park was the green of springtime. The last of the snow had disappeared two weeks ago and the cloudy weather of the past few days was no longer with us. I

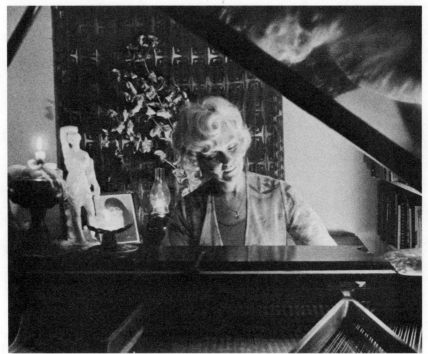

Sandy Solomon

lay down on the grass and it was surprisingly comfortable. I had to move around just a little to get the right curvature. I closed my eyes and tried to follow Dyveke's words, to let my body sink into the grass. As I became still, I could feel the sun beaming down on my face. I got visions of lying on a beach in the summer. I felt my whole body give way.

Then Dyveke was saying, "Pay attention to your body. What do you feel? Is one side more in contact with the ground? Do you feel tension? Let go of any portion of your body that feels tight. You want to practice becoming aware of your body. Many of you have holding patterns in parts of your body. You want to become able to sense these holding patterns. You also want to become aware of what it feels like when you totally relax these tense areas."

I felt a hand on my right shoulder. There was a gentle push and release and I realized that even though I was lying down and feeling pretty relaxed, my shoulders were a little tense. Another gentle push and release by the unseen hand, and I felt the tightness in my shoulders sink away.

"It is important in a Lifestyle Training Program to go within and listen. Learn to sense your body. Ask for guidance. Use mental pictures to get past difficult points in your training. The exercise we are doing now will help you begin to explore your innerspace.

"Now picture a sunstar about six inches above your head. Let's play with the star. Make it about the size of a dime. Move it out about ten feet. Now bring it back. Now make it larger, about the size of your hand, and change it into a square. Now make it a triangle. Swing it to the left. Now to the right."

It wasn't clear to me whether I was actually seeing the sunstar or not, but I could tell that it was about the size of a dime. When I imagined it being ten feet out, I had a sense of it being about that far away. For me it wasn't as if I were seeing a motion picture of the star, but yet it was there. When I swung it to the right, I felt that it was on my right. When I swung it to the left, I felt that it was to my left.

"Now collapse the star into a tiny point of light and bring it out about six inches in front of your face. Imagine another point of light at the bottom of your abdomen. Now connect these two points with a thin beam of light. Bring the beam up from your abdomen, through your stomach, along your windpipe, curving around your throat and out to the tiny point of light in front of your face."

At first, my mind wandered a bit. I thought of my youngest son who was supposed to play baseball this morning. I wondered if my secretary had finished typing the letters I had dictated yesterday. I remembered a credit card bill I had forgotten to pay. Then I recalled Dyveke talking about mind chatter, a perfect description of what was happening in my mind. But as I began to play with the beam of light, my mind became very still and focused. The intrusions of mind chatter began to lessen and then stopped all together.

"Now expand the beam of light and let it take the form of a tube extending from the bottom of the abdomen, up through your body and out in front of your face. Now imagine a tiny green ball at the top of the tube. As you breathe in, let the ball precede the rush of air all the way to the bottom of the tube. Then as you exhale, let the ball precede the rush of air all the way back up the top of the tube. Now just breathe easily for a bit, letting the ball go back and forth in the tube."

As I breathed in and out, pushing the ball down into my abdomen and then back up and out to the end of the tube, my body began to feel rather light. There was a warm glow all over. I began to feel a little as if I were floating. My mind was completely still. An incredible peacefulness came over me.

"Now extend the tube to a tree that is several hundred yards away, and as you exhale, imagine the ball being pushed through the tube all the way out to the tree. Then, as you inhale, imagine it being pulled back through the tube and into your body. After you have done this a few times, change the color of the ball. Let it be red. Now change it to purple as you exhale it and orange as you inhale it."

Purple out and orange in. Dyveke was talking. I was losing some of it. Green out. In the distance the sound of soft wind chimes, barely audible, coming in on a warm slow breeze. For some undetermined time I was completely out of awareness. Then back in for half a sentence. Then losing it again; my body becoming more like a gas than a solid and the parts floating lazily off in different directions. Then an instant when I'm no longer a separate entity. I don't know who I am, where I am, or what I am. Those questions don't even make sense. Is this what it means to be *at one with the universe*?

Now Dyveke is saying, "Lift your right leg up across your chest and let it fall over to your left side." Have I missed anything? I'm not quite with her but my right leg *is* bent over to my left side now. Dyveke continues with the instructions. I realize that we're doing some sort of exercise from this very relaxed state. Shoulders on the ground, head turned to the right. A spinal twist.

"Now imagine a point of white light just above your head. Imagine a second point above the head of the person on your right. Now connect these two points with a light streamer. Now feel the connection being made from person to person. You are tapped into that network now. Feel energy being circulated from person to person and back to you through the light streamer. Cause the energy to flow faster and faster through the circuit. Feel it radiating down through your body; through your head, shoulders, chest, abdomen, down each leg. Feel the group as one big energy system.

"If you have trouble visualizing the beam of light, make it shimmer." All of a sudden my beam of light becomes like a charged electrical wire with a white bolt of lightning surging around and around with ever-increasing speed. I begin to feel a connection with the person beside me even though I have no idea of who the person is or what he or she looks like.

"Now slowly open your eyes, but only partially. Keep a very soft focus. Roll over on your right side and slowly stand up, maintaining the soft focus with your eyes. Now pair up with someone near you. We're going to do about five minutes of slow running with a partner. Maintain the soft focus of your eyes and the calm, relaxed feeling that you have now for the duration of the run.

"As you run with your partner, imagine a small point of light in your abdomen and a small point of light in the abdomen of your partner. Connect these two points with a beam of light and pulsate energy back and forth between you and your partner. Maintain this connection throughout your run.

"As you run, project a streamer of light to a tree, a bush, a rock, or some other point in nature a hundred yards or so in the distance. Imagine this streamer being connected to a pulley at the tree or bush and feel yourself being pulled along to the tree or bush. Then at some point in your run, imagine yourself connected to a tiny white cloud that is sailing forward in the sky. Feel yourself being pulled up and forward by the momentum of the cloud. All the time, maintain the relaxed feeling and soft focus that you have now."

My partner and I started off on our slow run. I connected to her with the beam of light attached to my abdomen. As we ran, I sent a light streamer to the black bark of a tall tree in the distance. The tree began to spin around in position, winding the light streamer around and around its trunk and pulling me effortlessly along. Later I realized that the inner-space work we did this morning calmed my mind, took me through some stretching to prepare me to run, and helped me use visualizations to get energy both from my partner and from nature. I realize now that I wasn't running this morning: I was floating.

Chapter Five:
Awakening the
Feminine Principle

Turning Within and Listening

Many years ago, I discovered the power of using mental pictures to evoke physiological responses in my body. When playing tennis, I would *see* myself recovering deep backhand drives to the baseline by floating over the surface of the court. In skiing, I would glance down the projected fall line and *see* my hips wind up and uncurl as I gracefully "swished the hill."

Over the past years I have refined these processes in developing my training methods. I call this aspect of my work *innerspace*. In innerspace work we use mental imagery to "explore the unconscious by using the imagination under the direction of the conscious intellect and the will." Mental imagery techniques can play a valuable integrative role by bridging the conscious and unconscious as well as the rational and affective dimensions of our personality. It is these *innerspace* procedures combined with physical training that set my work apart from other methods.

Some innerspace techniques require a guide. I was the guide in the Toronto Workshop described earlier. Other techniques can be self-directed through imagination. Sometimes a tape recorder is used to dictate a procedure and play it back to oneself. Sometimes questions are formulated and answers are allowed to emerge as mental images: visualizations, pictures, dreamlike symbols; spontaneous messages from the unconscious.

89

I have conducted innerspace training on beaches and mountains while coaching athletes to compete in international races. I have used visualizations on injured athletes to help them improve the range of motion on a limb or joint. These techniques have stimulated a sense of team unity by helping members visualize connecting streamers of energy over a playing field and evoking a sense of unity and oneness. George Leonard and I have run pell-mell down a mountain visualizing "stepping into an infinite river of energy," flying at breakneck speeds, almost missing turns.

I have used these techniques to quiet an anxious client fraught with emotional distress, to inspire transcendent moments of inner awareness in high energy multi-media events for hundreds of people. I have even silently gone within to allow pictures to awaken my inner knowledge when coaching people on my morning runs, and have received information about clients who were injured or in distress. These techniques can be used anywhere, anytime, driving in a car, sitting in a meeting, playing tennis, making love. They are appropriate for every conceivable use of human experiencing.

These innerspace techniques have a variety of uses: to better understand our fears and drives, to get in touch with our conflicts, and to direct our energies in a more constructive way.

Taking time for *innerspace* work in your training schedule may seem frivolous or extravagant at first glance. It may seem silly to a beginning runner to "visualize yourself standing under a waterfall and allowing the rivulets of water to stream down your shoulders and back" in order to release your arm action. It may seem ridiculous to imagine that you are "coming down on soft air puffs" instead of hard pavement, so that your foot plant allows your skeletal muscle frame to descend gracefully with thousands of pounds of pressure on your metatarsal.

But you have not grown up in a culture or lifestyle that values the powers of the mind or the virtues of contemplative reflection, and it is natural that there is some resistance to seeing the value of innerspace work with physical training. Only recently has it come to be talked about in the media coverage of our sporting events. In your physical education classes you were never exposed to these processes.

In a mechanistic culture where power is defined by complex networks of finance and where the subtleties of human existence are often thought unworthy of serious consideration, the innerspaces of the artistic, questing part of yourself too often gives way to the practical realities of basic survival.

Knowledge is Within

In the human potential movement there is sometimes an urgent rush to

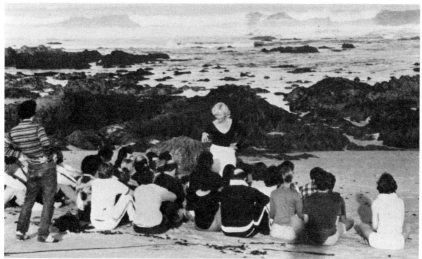

Sandy Solomon

experience a body of knowledge or methodology of self-improvement. Too many jump from teacher to teacher and guru to guru, hoping to find some remarkable tool or technique that has *the* answer for their lives. The ancient wisdom schools suggest a different path: one of turning within and listening, asking for guidance or using prayer. The implication is that all knowledge is contained within . . . in the *soul*.

> One method is a technique of "dialogue with the higher self." This is the practical application of the ancient and nearly universal belief that man has a higher aspect, or soul, and that this higher aspect can be contacted by the personality and asked for guidance. It consists of the assumption that within each of us is an endowment of wisdom, intuition, and sense of everyday life. The next step is to be in dialogue with it, trusting that it is there and it will answer." (From *Synthesis*: "The Realization of the Self," by Stuart Miller, Volume One, Number 2, 1975.)

The Hindus call this the *Atman*. Gandhi speaks of it as the "inner light of universal truth." It involves letting go of our identification with the analytical mind and liberating the creative aspects of our life that are often blocked. It is this right-brain, intuitive side, our feminine energy, that we want to bring to our Lifestyle Training Program.

Many athletes describe experiences that resemble mystical states in which all sense of personal limitation is dissolved into an oceanic feeling of universal cosmic consciousness.

Michael Murphy, the founder of Esalen Institute, after extensive research stemming from his longtime interest in the teachings of Sri Aurobindo and his study in India, compiled research that equated experiences athletes often had with the "Siddhis" or "special powers" acquired by mystics.

Awakening the Feminine Principle through Innerspace Work

It is ironic that every civilization that remains vital and alive to us today does so because of the passions of its artists, sculptors, musicians, poets — all in their time the most expendable members of their society. If we are to survive as a species, we must awaken the *feminine principle* in each of us, the principle that honors the soul of the artist. The feminine principle lies dormant beneath the external demands of making a living, keeping the house and car clean, and making sure we are not criticized because something is left undone. The feminine principle operates from the right hemisphere of the brain and reveals information from the unconscious mind.

In this chapter I am sharing with you some of the innerspace techniques and processes I use, and showing you how they have been used to awaken people to their feelings, to solve problems and overcome obstacles and negative self-programming, and even to improve times in a marathon. Sometimes innerspace work dramatically shatters a person's mode of functioning and results in a total reorganization of his or her life.

As a coach, an artist of the soul, I observe the quiet depths of fears and passions that erupt daily in the lives of people with whom I work. There are times when I feel I am a strange, undefined kind of healer, a shaman. Sometimes, in a circle, when people are lying with their heads together, I see tears stream quietly down the side of a cheek as I suggest they "feel the right and left side of their bodies." Going into innerspace releases a blockage of emotion, something no one was able to touch when it counted.

Physically training your body every day while also connecting to the hidden recesses of your collective "I" can change your life more quickly and dramatically than anything else you will experience . . . except a love-bond.

Innerspace techniques involve the use of active imagination, fantasy, guided imagery, visualization. Practice of these techniques can lead to an increased internal and external awareness. When combined with physical training, they allow you to control your physiological processes and transcend temporal limitations such as boredom, pain, injury, fear, self-doubt, worry, and stress, which in their slithering power deny the fullest expression of the total *I*.

Innerspace techniques allow you to condense and compress your accumulated experience, to get instant breakthroughs of incredible magnitude. Use of these techniques can enable you to unleash the intuitive, creative, artistic, feeling side of yourself that has too long been buried beneath layer upon layer of analytical, logical, statistical, left-brain living.

Benefits of Combining Innerspace Work with Physical Training.

There are many benefits that can accrue from combining innerspace work with training.

1. You will enjoy your training more because it becomes so fascinating. It becomes a joyous, playful, almost spiritual experience.

2. You will avoid injuries because you will be more aware of your body while training. Dr. William Brostoff, medical doctor and acupuncturist, once said: "Injuries happen when you are not 'awake'."

3. You will solve stressful personal and theoretical problems more easily because you will be able to short-circuit the "feedback tape loop system" of cause and effect and obtain input from the right hemisphere of your brain. You provide your bio-computer with fresh data and sometimes "instant breakthroughs."

4. You will feel revitalized *after* training because your creative imagination has been massaged by "playfulness."

5. You will have a deeper sense of internal beauty as the innerspace techniques extend your consciousness to other life forms. Your feelings will extend from personal ecology to planetary ecology to, perhaps, "cosmic connections." Certainly we live in an age in which extraterrestrial life is considered a distinct possibility.

6. As you eliminate the drudgery of training through the use of innerspace techniques, feelings of joy will spill over and create a gradual openness in your personality. You may find tendencies such as being overly compulsive, critical, impatient, withdrawn, slipping away and being replaced with a childlike expressiveness and compassion for others.

The power of the mind through the creation of visual images is only now coming to the forefront as a key factor both in healing and in training the will and intentionality.

There are numerous exercises you can use to begin to explore your innerspace. They all follow the same basic approach; after a few minutes of deep relaxation or autogenic work (such as self-hypnosis), allows a picture or mental image to appear. Then the image is allowed to permeate the body with emotional and sensing qualities.

The purpose of visualizations is to program the subconscious mind with some positive image, or reprogram the subconscious mind away from inappropriate thinking processes and instinctive responses, toward more positive processes and responses that are appropriate to the fullest functioning.

The following section is a compendium of innerspace techniques for your own exploration. The exercises are imaginative, free-flowing, sometimes outrageously "cosmic." When combined in a physical training program with the vast array of ways we can move, they are incredibly fascinating. Every artist evolves his or her own style, so it is up to you to put together a program of exercises that are appropriate to you. The important thing is not only to practice these exercises in your living room, but also to incorporate them in your physical training. The physical training of your body should be done while your mind is relaxed. These exercises will help you relax your mind and keep it relaxed during training. You will learn to tune in to your subconscious mind and intuitive wisdom, and will become more aware of your moods and feelings, so that you can start to expand your faculties to reach higher levels of consciousness.

Innerspace Exercises

These preliminary exercises dampen the left hemisphere of the brain and allow the intuitive right hemisphere to release information stored in your subconscious mind. Use them to learn to concentrate and focus while lying on the floor in your room. Then use them when you are running or swimming to train your mind as you train your body.

The key to innerspace work is *relaxation*, so the tone of the environment should be soothing and inspirational. You want a trusting environment where you feel no threat of intrusion. Be sure to unplug your phone. You want a loving atmosphere that is aesthetic, with flowers, soft lights, incense. You may want to play some music that is restful and elevating to your spirit. You want your senses to be stimulated and heightened.

Unbuckle your belt, remove your shoes, be warm and comfortable. Sit in a chair or lie on the floor with eyes closed and palms up. Don't be overly fatigued. Eat lightly beforehand and don't use alcohol prior to this work because it may put you to sleep. Don't worry if at first you *do* go in and out of a sleep state. This is normal and gradually diminishes.

Start to breathe deeply, allowing all the fatigue of the day to float away. Begin to feel a reverence for a unique, personal encounter with your subconscious: a sense of "personal honoring of the self." Be positive.

Now you are ready to try one or more of the following exercises.

1. *Ask for guidance.* You can use prayer or invocation to your higher consciousness, to the collective unconscious, or to a spiritual source. Feel a sense of relinquishing control to the universal force that created you.

2. *Reduce anxieties, doubts, and worries.* For example, use Robert Mon-

roe's technique of imagining a metal box in which you will place all of your cares, worries, anxieties, undone deeds, etc. Then close the heavy metal lid on the box. Or picture your cares and worries being floated away in a balloon, or burned in a fire in a meadow.

3. *Cleanse your body with light.* Send light streamers through your body to all parts and feel internally lighted and cleansed.

4. *Become aware of your body through internal scanning.* Mentally get in touch with body parts such as the back of your knees, holding patterns in your shoulders, hips. Sense your right and left sides and determine if there is a difference. Sense the alignment of your feet, the turn-out of your ankles, and follow that alignment up through your knees and hips. Sense how this internal awareness can affect your movement. Visualize yourself running or playing your sport with this awareness.

5. *Heighten your suggestibility.* Visualize the numbers 1 to 10 on a blackboard and count them. Descend in an elevator going from 24th floor to the first. Count the floors as you go down. Walk down a spiral staircase and count down the steps. These exercises will dampen the left hemisphere of your brain, your mind chatter and logical thought, and allow you to relax into an altered state of consciousness which is essential in exploring innerspace. Some call this the *alpha* state.

6. *Get in touch with your immediate feeling state.* Think about the emotions of love, compassion, hate, jealousy, and see where they register in your body. Switch your feeling states. You'll see that you have the capacity to control what you are feeling. You don't have to be overwhelmed by negative emotions because of someone else's behavior. Learning to take responsibility for what you are experiencing is a key to personal wholeness, and is necessary if you are to reach your highest potential.

   Place yourself in situations which evoke various feeling states and watch yourself react. Get into it fully. If you are thinking of *hate* or *jealousy*, really work it up. Sense it in your body. Then switch your emotions.

7. *Review events of day.* Credit yourself with positives; reprogram negatives. Replay the negatives in your mind the way you would choose to handle them now.

8. *Focus attention.* Imagine a dot of white light in the center of your forehead. Expand and contract it. Elongate it into a bar. Extend it around your head as a loop. Turn it into a circle. Shrink it to a dot. Take it into the center of your head and then to different parts of your body. Now extend the dot. There is a whole horizon of tools built around this exercise that you can use in running, swimming, biking, skiing, even racket sports, to focus attention, keep thoughts positive, and improve performance, internal relaxation, and joy.

9. *Transfer energy and solve problems.*   Focus on a tiny white dot and send it mentally to an object in the room. Contract it again to a dot. Send it as an energy streamer to another person, with you or far away. Enlarge the dot and place the consciousness of someone you love inside. Peer into their eyes. Send loving energy. Extend the dot to an energy network connecting several people. Sense a tree. Send a streamer outside to the tree and wrap it around a branch. Play imagine. If you are not are not sure it's happening, pretend. Act *as if* you are seeing the tiny white dot from the center of your forehead bringing the awareness of others into your consciousness. Convey thoughts telepathically.

   Place a difficult problem inside the enlarged dot, charge it with imaginary energy, and dissolve it. Put the solution you desire in its place.

10. Sensing your energy body.   Outline your physical body with a second body, your *energy body* or aura. This is the subtle electromagnetic field surrounding the body that can now be detected by Kirlian photography.

   As you lie on the floor, use a white light to make a mental outline of your physical body. Take about three minutes to do this. Any parts you can't find, aren't aware of, that feel "foreign" may be areas where you have an injury.

   After you have traced your body map, visualize a white dot in the center of your forehead. Charge it up. Make it very very bright. Now send it down and through and over your body map and into your internal organs. Allow any pictures you sense to float across your consciousness.

   Now begin to play with this body map or energy body. Extend your light to six inches around you; to one foot around you; to the ceiling, through the floor, to the roof, and to others in the room. Change the colors of the light to red, green, blue, purple. See what you sense and feel.

   Imagine you can place your consciousness six inches above you and can look down at yourself.

11. *Healing with visualizations.*   Irving Oyle, in *The Healing Mind*, says, "The ancients believed that the key to healing (wholeness) lay in the mental image. In order to induce formation of the mental image, it is necessary to go into a meditative state which turns off the thinker. When the left hemisphere is at rest or in alpha, it is possible to reprogram the computer by means of the conscious image of the healthy state. This image is transmitted holographically and reproduced in the matter of the body."

By now some of you may be asking, "How in the world can I do anything as crazy as 'sense my energy body' or heal with visualizations?" I can appreciate your consternation. But my experience is full of examples where, often to my complete amazement, even the simplest of innerspace techniques has made a dramatic difference. I have seen people overcome inertia and find the motivation to begin a training program, eliminate repeated injuries to a muscle or limb, or, in the case of a nationally ranked athlete, surpass his wildest ambition. Again, just as *starting to move* is the key to physical training, *starting to allow* is the key to innerspace training.

Innerspace and Running

Visualizing during physical training can greatly enhance your body's ability to relax and *flow* with movement. The following are images you can use with running.

Sky-hook   Imagine you are being elevated and lifted upward and that your body is dangling loosely and freely. Pretend you are a "skeleton blowing in the wind."

Bamboo shoot   Image your neck as a shoot of bamboo gently resting between your shoulders. This releases your arm action.

Waterfall   Visualize a stream of water flowing down your back and streaming off your shoulders. This visualization helped a novice marathoner complete his first race in 90-degree heat.

Golden tube   Mentally picture a golden tube connecting the back of your throat to your abdomen. Imagine your breath as a golden ball going up and down inside the tube. Fully expand that tube with each breath so that it becomes a cavern. Allow your breath to go deeper into your abdomen.

Pools of water   Sense pools of water around your knees to absorb the shockwave of each foot plant. Release all ligament and tendon bindings around knee socket: such bindings are a common cause of injury.

Air puffs   Imagine each foot coming down on a soft air puff and, with awareness, that you are rolling from heel to toe lightly on the outside of your foot.

Giant hand   When running up a hill, visualize a giant hand pushing you along so that you are propelled by a source of energy not your own.

Light streamers   Extend your energy, in the form of a streamer, from a small white dot in your forehead to a distant tree, rock, telephone pole. Hook it around the object and imagine the streamer being wound onto a pulley and yourself being drawn effortlessly to the object.

Soft eyes   Run with your eyes partially closed. This allows your intuitive sense to open. It also releases part of the lower spine. Look about 30 feet in front of you. Don't drop your head to look at the ground, as this puts your body out of alignment. Allow your feet to find their own way.

Running with a partner Imagine a streamer of energy connecting your shoulders with your partner's. Take turns being in the lead and being equal. This dance of energy exchange breaks down patterns of power.

Running with a group Let each member of the group visualize a sunstar over his or her head and send out light streamers to hook onto that imaginary sunstar. This sets up an energy field and can actually pull along the weakest members of the group without strain or injury. It can create a sense of joy and inner connectedness among members of the group.

In addition, you can use imagery such as a phalanx, feeling like birds flying in formation or sled dogs running in a team. I sometimes suggest that a running phalanx continually change positions to become aware of our interdependence and the subtle energy forces about us. Accelerating and slowing down, swerving and running backwards, a group can manage to work together just like birds or sled dogs.

Play with your environment Visualize a small dot of iridescent white light spinning in your forehead. Then loop it around your head and project it onto living things at a distance, such as a tree. Feel the energy of the tree and let that energy pull you toward it.

Look at a delicate leaf. Feel its fragility, its vulnerability. Run to the leaf, touch it gently, go inside.

Imagine a deer running at your side. Connect your energy with the grace of the deer and *become* the deer as you run. Step inside its body and float through your run. Jim Waste, a nationally ranked masters runner, used this image extensively while running marathons.

Imagine you are an Indian running in complete silence over the soft grass, as if the people you pass could neither see nor hear you. Let the wind gently push you along, the sun fill your body with soft, golden energy.

Become leaf and grow with branch. Look into the eyes of an animal and feel its soul. Allow the song of a bird to ripple through your muscles as you run. Know the ultimate oneness of all things.

When the psyche connects to other living things, you begin to accept your own process of evolution, your own metamorphosis. It is astounding how little it takes to shake loose people's psyches from where they are stuck. It is as if a miracle of instant growth transforms negative, self-destructive tendencies to heights of personal power. A miracle is a condensation and compression of time. Miracles come in a state of miracle-mindedness. If you accept that your life is a miracle, you can transcend your time-space reality.

In the following sections, I am including some *vignettes* to illustrate how these techniques can be applied. It captures the *poetic quality* of this work.

Running Past the "Sphinx"

Training time can be a time of inspiration. It can be used for intuitive break-throughs in problem solving. You can playfully use props from nature as your cues.

An early morning run prompted this experience with radio producer/announcer Bill Gordon.

> As we ran down the beach, Bill said to me: "Dyveke, can you believe that 15 years ago I weighed 195 lbs, hated everyone, drank booze, and fucked around in that whole crazy TV-radio world of mine? I've had stations in San Francisco. I've had interview talk shows for seven years and celebrities have swept in and out of my home. But now I've become a *health nut*. All I can do is talk about nutrition, diet, running, and a different kind of personal medicine."

> As we talked, mile after mile of the beach unfolded to our slow steps. We did the usual things of letting the shoulders go, opening up the chest, exhaling, coming down lightly on the back of the heel, rolling on the outside of the foot. We jogged under the pier and through a barnacled area. Looking at the beach, I said: "Bill, it's like an undulating soundwave. Watch how the water is going back to the sand and pulling water out of the sand. I can hear music as I look at that! And down the beach, look at the lifeguard tower through the fog. It's like a Sphinx overlooking the ocean. If we had a particular problem to solve, we could create a mental image while running down this vibrating sound wave of wet sand. Information would come into our consciousness, giving us insight into our problem. Let's try it."

> Bill was a little astounded at this idea but liked the originality. So we ran down the beach as one perfect energy field. Every step, every breath, the hair along our arms moved in complete unison. With every movement of our rippling spines, the Sphinx came closer to us. I closed my eyes and imagined I was in Egypt, running over the desert. But even more important, I had an intuitive flash about Bill. During the run I had been teaching Bill how to run with soft eyes to awaken his sensing abilities. I had a distinct image while beaming energy to the lifeguard tower that Bill should be doing exactly what I was doing, some kind of coaching.

Soft Eyes

Later Bill talked about how he'd like to teach blind people to jog. "I see so many blind people at the beach and I'd like to turn them on to running." Within weeks he had a Sunday morning "Run With Bill." He quit his job in radio and is now a New Age Coach in nutrition and fitness. Two years later he wrote the following article for *PreventionM;*.

> We are jogging along the beach in San Diego when Dyveke Spino, the fantastic physical fitness coach, says, "Now, make soft eyes." This, she explains, means letting the eyelids relax and nearly close. You can still

see through the slits, but the scene suddenly becomes one of softness and restfulness and lacks strong definition. I once read about the tremendous amount of energy required to just see, so it came as no surprise that closing my eyes would really conserve energy.

One day, I decided to go one step further in the *soft eyes* approach. If almost closing the eyes could make one feel relaxed, how much better would it be if I could close them all the way? Running along the water's edge, in the hard sand, you can see far into the distance and notice any obstructions that might be in your path. I picked a place with about 100 yards of nice, smooth sand stretching out ahead. I went *soft eyes* and then went all the way.

Suddenly, for the first time in my life, I ran with no vision! It was an eerie feeling in the beginning; one of slight fear of where to put my feet and "Am I veering to the right or left?" Every 50 feet or so there was a compulsion to open my eyes a bit and see just where I was stepping. But during those moments of jogging with my eyes closed, I felt an increased sense of awareness of what my entire body was doing: how my head was held, my shoulders, where my feet were — and all those proper alignments that seem so difficult to imagine with the eyes open. I knew I was on to something.

I invited Art Durson, a blind friend, to go jogging with me on the beach. We used a long, light plastic pole and I led as we took off down the beach. He loved it, and after a while I got the idea that even without the guiding pole, directions can be given verbally by the sighted person to the other one, such as "a little to the left . . . steady . . . now a little to the right."

A number of things can come out of all this. One is developing an unusual trust in the person who guides. Another is the exalted feeling of turning one's self over completely to the sensations of nature and a new awareness of one's body. A bonus is the sense of storing up energy engendered by the oxygen intake and the aerobic effect of jogging. And, of course, you can do this with a friend who is not blind. Get a good friend, someone you can trust, and head for a nice stretch of sandy beach, or perhaps a clean grassy surface that is good and flat. Go *soft eyes* then go all the way. Relax your shoulders, hands and wrists . . . nice and straight now . . . a little to the left . . . now steady . . ." (From "A New Vista: Blind Jogging" in *Prevention* magazine.)

Speed Training and Shades of Green

Mel is a 50-year-old lawyer who just started running a year ago. He had laid the long slow distance base and was now ready for more advanced techniques in interval and oxygen debt training. By pushing his body to its limits over short distances with spaces for recovery, and repeating this cycle with varying distances of 20 to 150 yards, his ability to endure stress loads would be increased. This experience on Mt. Tamalpais happened the day he started speed work.

Today Mel started speed work. The silver-gray light shone into the pools of water to the side of the track; the full moon lent its mystical light and the sun's rays sent warmth to our mittened hands. We started with warm-up and yoga stretches. Today the cycle was to bring tempos and rhythms into the life of Mel Morgan.

We had been talking business and I wanted to cleanse his mind of all deliberations. As my hand lay across his shoulder I could to feel his day already descending into the sinews of his muscles, the slight hump coming across his shoulder from too many pressures and time deadlines.

As my eyes swept across the colors of green, I said, "Now start to look at all the different shades in front of you, the light green grass, the delicate blue-gray of the eucalyptus trees, the deep, dark, green-shadowed pine trees. Start to appreciate all the different colors and flow of the green and allow those different rhythms and colors to start coming into your body, down through your spine, streaming down like ripples of energy: green, light green, blue-green and dark green. This will be the way you feel as you start to move through the rhythms and tempos of the speed work."

We started with a slow warm-up and build-up, gradually accelerating. I said, "Mel, stay right on my left shoulder and think of that low foot plant, coming down softly on the light green energy streamer that's going through your body."

As we started to do another build-up and get into a 30-40 percent acceleration, I said, "Now the green is shifting to a blue-green. Start to lift the arms and pull with the sun, exhaling the breath and lifting the knees high and just sailing out over the light green into the blue-green."

As we rounded the bend, we started into a 60 percent build-up. It's like a soundwave, starting with a shake-up, going into the shuffle, leading with the knees, and then pulling the arms and lilting over the ground. I could see Mel did not have a natural sense of sprinting, of just taking off with his body and allowing the upper torso to relax, but he did respond to the visual image of the green streamers of energy coursing through his body.

At the straight-away, I said, "Mel, try to imagine that blue-green eucalyptus tree clearly in your mind. And now, as my hand has found your back, imagine that tree coming right into your body." Almost automatically, the hump in his back began letting up. We did a fresh sprint down the track. At the far end he imagined a wire running from his abdomen and to a large pulley attached to a tree at the other end. As he ran the next straight-away, the pulley of energy from the tree was winding him up.

So Mel had his first speed lesson with the shades of green on the horizon, visualizing eucalyptus trees coming through his body, and being connected to a tree by an energy streamer winding him toward the tree as he lifted his knees and sailed down the straight-away.

Using Visualizations and Body Sensing in Other Sports

The breadth of application of innerspace techniques to sports is almost limitless.

Tennis Flow

Tennis is the fastest-growing sport in the world. I wanted to bring a different awareness to the teaching and practice of this sport. As I became involved in creating the Esalen Sports Center and saw the possibility of using sports and games for *self-awareness and inner perfection*, I took another look at how tennis was being played and taught. I also reflected on my many years as a competitive athlete and tennis pro. There is something fundamentally wrong when a beautiful, graceful sport such as tennis is twisted to serve the interest of high finance through expensive clubs and dues, and ceases to serve the greatest need of our culture, which is to *train our bodies and our consciousness to higher levels of personal growth and transcendence*.

It seemed to me that much tennis being played was causing thousands to suffer needless tennis elbow, strained shoulders, twisted knees, and lower back difficulty. I also saw the severe psychological stress, anxiety, and lowered self-esteem that permeated many competitive tennis circles, especially those for teen-age players. I saw the need to teach tennis in such a way as to introduce the emerging healing modalities that developed balance, alignment, flexibility, and inner power, along with developing the powers of the mind.

Blending concentration exercises with visualizations and mental imagery is the essence of *Tennis Flow*, which I taught for five years at Esalen Sports Center through workshops, clinics, and university courses.

George Leonard, author of *The Ultimate Athlete*, describes his reintroduction to tennis using my methods:

> I had not held a racket in my hands for over five years when I went out recently to sample the new approach to tennis instruction as offered by Dyveke Spino, one of its leading exponents.
>
> Dyveke, a flamboyant Scandinavian blonde who has been a ski instructor and concert pianist as well as a tennis pro, teaches a version of the game she calls "Tennis Flow." Her approach begins with rigorous attention to weight training and aerobic conditioning; she believes that thousands of Americans are injuring their arms, elbows, backs, and necks through lack of conditioning and jerky, overly-aggressive movements. As we walked onto the courts, she pointed out players who were fighting the ball, force against force, shoulders raised, arm muscles rigid and tense.
>
> After my long layoff, I was shocked at the amount of aggression I could sense all around me . . . the grim, tight-jawed faces, the muttered curses, the rackets almost hurled into the net. Had my perceptions changed or was there actually an increase in this poorly veiled hostility? I recalled a recent conversation with a friend. "What I really love about tennis," she told me, "is that I can spend an hour cramming the ball down my opponent's throat and then sit on the terrace drinking Pimm's Cup with him after the game. That's civilization at its best."
>
> Our session began with meditation. Dyveke called upon the metaphor of a star of light above each of our heads:

"Close your eyes," she told me, "and think of the light above your head as flowing through your entire body, filling your body with light, then expanding to join the two of us." We were to meditate on our court as being a calm pool of energy. "No matter how turbulent the energy is on the other courts, our court is still and serene at all times."

Just as this image was coming clear to me, there was a sharp, choked-off expletive from an adjacent court and the metallic clatter of a racket striking the ground. For a moment I questioned the wisdom of sitting with eyes closed in this place of flying objects.

It was not until the next exercise that I achieved the serenity my teacher had in mind. Eyes open and soft now, we moved around within our court (a calm, still pool) as ripples of radiant light. Maintaining this image, we practiced lateral movements along the baseline. Then we stood there, and Dyveke had me imagine myself at the apex of a triangle. An angled step to the right or to the left would take me to the imaginary triangle's other two corners. Between my two hands I held an imaginary bowl of water about four feet in diameter. I stepped to the right corner of the triangle and swung the bowl to the left in a way that spilled the water evenly over its edge. That gentle, liquid movement was to be the foundation of my forehand. Stepping to the left corner of the triangle and swinging the bowl in the other direction allowed me to gain the feeling of a flowing, liquid backhand.

At last, Dyveke offered me a tennis racket. She taught me to hold it gently, as one would hold a living bird. Only at the instant of impact with the ball would my hand tighten on the racket, and then it would relax again. Here, my teacher turned to her musical experience to explain how a pianist can achieve force and majesty in the same manner, keeping the wrists entirely loose and relaxed except at the precise moment of impact.

She let me take a few practice swings, then went to the other side of the net and began throwing me easy balls.

"Don't think about where the ball's going," she told me. "Don't think about anything . . . just that smooth flow, like you're spreading water out of a bowl."

By now I was indeed flowing with her words and had little difficulty swinging easily. Gradually, it occurred to me that almost all my shots were clearing the net perfectly. She threw balls to my backhand, and I continued swinging easily; there seemed no difference between backhand and forehand. I surrendered to the rhythm of the experience. The sounds and motions in the other courts fell from my awareness.

It was all so effortless that I suddenly found myself quite surprised. And here was that topspin I had previously coveted and pursued. I began congratulating myself and imagining future success on the courts. My energy rose from my *hara* to my chest. I began hitting shots into the net.

"You're doing fine," Ms. Spino told me. "Just don't think and don't plan."

"You're so right," I said.

Gradually my teacher guided me back into the delightful state of *not doing* that had allowed me to do so well. That being enough for a first lesson, she went on to explain and demonstrate further applications of the energy dimension in developing net play, the lob, the serve. What most fascinated me was the way she envisaged competitive play. She suggested the possiblity of considering the person on the other side of the net not as your opponent but as your partner. In this context, a well-hit ball becomes a gift of energy, freely delivered. The gift may be returned, then exchanged again and again, linking the two players in a single energy field. The breathing of the two can be synchronized, with each player exhaling as the ball leaves the racket and inhaling upon its return.

Does this mean that you always hit your ball to the other player's strong side so that it is more likely to be returned? Far from it. In actual play, you hit the ball to your "partner's" weakness, to the undeveloped area of the energy field, and you expect the same. Thus both of you have the opportunity to achieve more of your potential, and the total field between you is strengthened.

You might also become a "winner," which could be all to the good. But I can't help thinking that there are ways of keeping score that don't appear on the sports pages. And I can't quite bring myself to believe that the grace, centeredness, and verve . . . or the rigidity and anger . . . we learn on the court is entirely left behind in the locker room. As much as we try to ignore our bodies, they are always with us. They *are* us.

A typical *tennis flow* workshop begins with the participants sitting in a circle. I lead them into deep relaxation, while having them pay attention to their breathing.

In a soft voice, I begin: "Imagine a picture of the ideal athlete you choose to be. Surround that picture with the consciousness you desire and step into that body. Enter a meadow and flow over the ground, effortlessly doing the rhythms and tempos of cardiovascular training. Now shift these images to a tennis court and interchange the feelings of being in the meadow with stroking a ball from the baseline. First move slowly and then gradually accelerate. Sense your body unwinding gracefully with impact and centered power. As speeding balls enter your *force field of light* at various angles, feel your body responding with grace, power, extreme joy.

"Sense your body pivoting around an ignited vertebra, your hips a fluidly rotating lazy susan, as you bring energy up through the arms and shoulders into the stroke."

At this point, the class moves onto the court in a state of deep relaxation to combine visualizations with the actual physical movements. "On the base line, with spine relaxed and mind calm, superimpose the meadow image over the court. Slowly begin stroking. Then accelerate the pace, angle, placement. Inhale as your partner hits and exhale through the stroke. The knees are springs as the body moves effortlessly to position. Visualize the trajectory of the ball *before* the stroke as each of you works in his or her own personal innerspace to keep your mental images positive, powerfully centered, and your body relaxed."

To teach the serve, I show people how to visualize and imprint the distance between the ball's leaving the hand and the height it must be hit to come *over* the ball. They rehearse this over and over with a racket swing, without the ball. Then it is rehearsed visually. Next, they do it without the ball or racket, but as body movement with eyes closed. Finally, it's all put together. Many people have hitches in their movements or throw the ball too far forward or backwards. It is only when they become *aware* of what they have been doing kinesthetically and through mental imagery that they can change it. I then teach people to whip the spine, allowing energy to go up and out through the body into the stroke, reaching upwards without any inhibition to the natural movement. The serve is the testing ground, too often, of one's self-image and confidence. I find that when people *flow* on the tennis court, they tend to move more fluidly in accepting themselves and others.

When you play the net, it's so fast that you must repond in every direction, kinesthetically and instinctively. Your other senses take over. I teach people to visualize themselves as a *hummingbird*, even 200-pound males! As I told Ron, "You want to sense and feel yourself still and quiet, yet able to dart and move in any direction at will. Tension, release, tension, release. Don't hold the racket tightly and burn unnecessary energy. Be calm, dart, relax, center." Along with these techniques I teach various Feldenkrais exercises to limber the feet, ankles, shoulder and wrists beforehand. (See Chapter 7 on flexibility.)

In sum:

When playing tennis, the energy of our bodies should become a musical instrument. To train the body, don't go out with locked arms and locked muscles. Don't go bent on making a personal statement against the elements. Train the body as a beautiful, delicate, lilting instrument. Use rhythms, tempos, asymmetrical movements. Burst with percussion, speed, and explosion. Then recoil to a quiet, meditative state. Play your body like Mozart.

Concentration and Golf

Concentration is the key to the game of golf. The mental ability to direct images with clear focusing is crucial to practice. *Tratak*, steady gazing at a particular point or object without blinking, develops concentration and mental focusing.

Candle Gazing. Keep a candle flame three to four feet away from your body. The level of your eyes and the candle flame should be in a horizontal line. Sit erect, keeping the spine straight and the body relaxed. For one minute look at the flame with a steady gaze and without blinking. Then close the eyes, relax the eye muscles, and visualize the flame between the eyebrows for a minute. Then again gaze with open eyes on the flame. After a minute, relax and close your eyes. Continue this process for five or six minutes. Gradually increase the period of gazing from one to three minutes, spending equal time relaxing the eyes. This exercise stimulates the nerve centers, has a soothing effect on cranial nerves, encourages concentration, i.e., enables the mind to become one-pointed, and strengthens the eyes.

A golf professional describes an innerspace technique he uses before every shot. He calls it "Going to the Movies."

> I never hit a shot, even in practice, without having a very sharp, in-focus picture of it in my head. It's like a color movie. First I *see* the ball in the precise place I want it to finish, nice and white and lying up high on the bright green grass. Then the scene quickly changes and I *see* the ball going there: its path, trajectory and shape, even its behavior on landing. Then there's a sort of fade-out and the next scene shows me making the kind of swing that will turn the previous images into reality. Only at the end of this short, private Hollywood spectacular do I select a club and step up to the ball.

Handling Hostile Energy

If you are subject to temper outbursts, severe self-criticism, or aggressive or stressful environments, visualize yourself as a *sieve* and allow hostile or negative energy to pass through your body. Mentally rehearse agitation in an environment such as noise, yelling crowds, wind, etc., and visualize yourself as calm and concentrated in a pool of light. Strong evocative statements affirming the will, such as "I will be calm, centered, lighted, as I trust in my ability to play to my maximum effort with keen concentration" tends to substitute positive for negative images.

Avoiding Injuries and Survival Situations

Dr. Lee Pulos, a Canadian psychotherapist, uses innerspace training in coaching athletes. He once trained a world-class race car driver to turn off his ignition switch automatically if he crashed. Failure to do this is the leading cause of death in auto-racing accidents. He also found that a volleyball team of national Canadian rank did phenomenally better if the players practiced visualizing their plays during regular practice sessions.

While I was at Strathcona Lodge on Vancouver Island, my colleague and friend Barbara Coffman went on a backpacking trip with four others into the wilds of the rugged Canadian back country. The leader of the group, a seasoned mountaineer, suffered a dislocated shoulder while repelling off a ledge. It was imperative that the rest of the group execute this particular maneuver and Barbara began assisting the others. While so doing, she suffered an injured knee. Another girl in the party, owing to the tension of being unfamiliar with the outdoors, exhibited a minor nervous breakdown. In this state of crisis two members of the party decided to hike out to get a rescue plane and Barbara was left to meet it. The leader and the other girl were in pain and shock.

Barbara managed to walk ten hours on her injured knee to meet the plane and guide them to the party. She told me upon returning to the Lodge, "Dyveke, it was all the training in visualization and positive affirmations we have done that kept me alive and hopeful. That trail became lighted with pulleys and sunstars as I sent healing energy to my knee and to other members of the party."

Innerspace training, I'm sure, calms and allows more centered decisions when caught in a survival crises such as Barbara's.

Imprinting Relaxation

Innerspace work can be blended with spinal flexibility exercises and sensing to imprint a feeling of relaxation while mentally rehearsing specific movements in a sport. This approach was used at the University of California, Davis, in May of 1976. About 60 college students were involved in an array of sports: skiing, tennis, basketball, track and field (javelin). Many spoke privately of injuries and hang-ups. I improvised free-flowing visualizations to imprint a different "body sense" while rehearsing relaxation techniques.

> An athlete needs to use the body with impact and force, yet at the same time in harmony. If you are going to ski at 30-60-70 mph through a blizzard or down a steep slope through slalom gates, you've got to let your knees go through the gates while the body unwinds at the same time. You've got to hold an edge. You've got to watch the plant of a pole and know when to lift it up. You've got to know when to go with the mountain. You can improve your performance by visualizing these movements in a relaxed state.

> If you are going to play tennis, you have to know how to charge up to the net but not overhit the ball, or hit it with locked muscles. You have to know how to use tension, power, compression, and impact with balance and deep relaxation. The way to train is to play with the body in a state of deep relaxation. Sense and visualize your movements away from the pull of gravity.

> The javelin throw is a primordial explosion, a supreme single effort. You can visualize an energy streamer or a bolt of lightning. Charge, holding the lightning bolt, release it, yell, unwind your spine, whip your hips and explode.

> In basketball, float over the court, quiet your mind, still the body as it works with maximum effort. Say to yourself, "I'm just an air puff, floating up into the air." Sense yourself and teammates joined as a moving energy field and visualize light streamers. Send thoughts during the play. Allow your consciousness an incredible range of fantasy and you will find your total body responding with joyous energy and efficiency.

Innerspace techniques such as guided fantasies, imagery, and meditation calm the mind and take the athletic experience to other realms. Creative visualizations stimulate the imagination and seem to allow the discovery or creation of a unifying center of the self. My methods seem to aid in training concentration and developing the will by focusing thoughts towards the execution of a goal. Evocative imagination practiced before or combined with sport endeavors is a powerful tool to set off a chain of motor reactions that use skeletal muscles with balance and harmony.

Innerspace and Swimming

Swimming is an excellent physical activity in which to combine various physical tempos and rhythms with visualizations to train the will and stimulate the imagination. It is possible to use visualizations in your swimming program to help you overcome negative habits, recover from injuries, improve self-image, solve problems, and connect to inspirational moments of awareness. The following are some examples.

Using Affirmations While Swimming

First, do four laps; long, slow, gliding, freestyle. Then rest. While in the water, close your eyes and visualize a golden ball in the center of your forehead. Make it sparkling and radiant. Allow feeling to flow through your body. Expand the golden ball and send streamers of energy across the pool and back.

Now clearly place the picture of the body you desire in the golden ball and swim, holding the image. Swim as if you are already in that body. Allow a series of pictures that depict things in your lifestyle that need altering to flow into your consciousness.

Now swim one or two fast laps in another stroke (back stroke or breast stroke, for example) with real determination and power, repeating to yourself one or more positive affirmations you have decided on before your swim.

Here are some affirmations that one of my students, Laura, used:

> I, Laura, deeply desire to train twice a week.

> I, Laura, will discipline my will to guide me in the self-management of my endurance training.

> I, Laura, am becoming stronger and healthier. I am transcending my limitations. I believe in myself and trust myself.

> I, Laura, deserve self-love and physical well-being.

Interspecies Communication

I was spending the summer in Santa Barbara and swimming to the pier almost every day. One day I had been reading Carl Sagan's *Cosmic Consciousness* while sunbathing, and was astounded by the implications that more advanced civilizations, billions of years old, might have species attempting "interterrestrial communication."

Having worked with John Lilly and Robert Monroe in attempting to develop my consciousness for such communication, I felt it was possible that I could, with proper discipline, develop altered states of consciousness that would help me get a glimpse of such possibilities.

As I entered the water, I thought, "My God, perhaps we *can* connect to other species. John Lilly has been successful, in part, with dolphins. And Robert Monroe has done so by recording volumes of material from a source of such incredible supra-intelligence that it mocks our civilization (See the References). Today I'm going to try to visualize in an effort to bring about such communication."

About an hour and a half into the swim, I was literally trying to send out an energy streamer to an imaginary dolphin. And something incredible happened. A sea otter popped up and started to swim with me. Yes! At that precise moment, I saw the back of a head that I thought was a skin diver. As it turned around, I saw it had whiskers. I was startled and yelled. The otter dived. I continued the swim.

A few minutes later, the otter appeared again and started diving all about me, as if playing with me. I started to laugh and said, "Oh, my friend, come and swim with me. You are so beautiful . . ." Then the idiocy hit me. "He can't understand what I'm saying. I'll have to communicate telepathically through *energy*." I sent loving thoughts and asked him questions about the sea. As I did so, I let random pictures come into my mind. All the way to the pier, the otter darted just close enough to swish my leg. Once my arm came down on his back.

I was able to see the tiny opening for hearing. I peered directly into the black depths of his eyes and the funny mouth that looks as if it is smiling. The immense humor of the incident hit me when I reached the pier. A stream of people, following this unpremeditated "water act" were lined up and taking pictures. One Italian fisherman leaned way over the pier and said: "Don't worry lady, he won't bite." Opening my eyes through the vaseline and hat that squished my face, I replied, "Yes, but how does he know I won't bite him?"

As soon as I left the range of the pier, the otter joined me again. This time we were "grooving." With my strokes and his dives, we were moving along down the Santa Barbara coastline with an amused audience following us. We didn't care. I finally had my long-awaited swimming partner.

Now, whether my *thoughts* had anything to do with evoking this exchange, we will never know. But, according to some highly renowned scientists, it is a possibility. I had been fasting, and had so cleansed and detoxified my body that all my senses were much clearer.

I am not proposing that these visualizations and innerspace techniques will enable you to communicate with the animal kingdom or extraterrestial intelligence. But many of you have animals you feel "attuned" to. Carl Sagan's work points out that the arrogance of our human condition must give way to a love of all life and a belief in our interdependence. The first step is to awaken our finer sensitivities to nature.

Echo Lake, Capturing the Magic Moments

An experience at Echo Lake seems to capture the subtle power of all the things I've shared in this chapter on innerspace. Echo Lake is a jewel, tucked beside Desolation Valley in the Sierras of California, elevation 7,500 feet. There are no roads or electricity, just a peaceful haven with only a few sailboats and an occasional motorboat. I was visiting my friend, Jeanne Gibbs.

> I had spent the previous August morning on a ten-mile run, past the lakes, up over the rocks, darting on my toes, sprinting down the forest paths, stepping over the snow patches, and passing the hikers up the steep, rocky grades to Desolation Valley. I knew the power in my body and at times even picked my way down the slopes like a goat, to graze in blue shadows dancing around granite cliffs. Sometimes I ran as a displaced animal, opening my pores to the infinite power around me.
>
> Today I wanted to swim across the lake. "Dyveke, you're crazy. Nobody has ever swum across the lake. It was pure melted ice just three weeks ago." "I know, Jeanne, but I can take cold water and I would like to do it." So I put some oil on my skin, put on my suit and hat, tucked the pink foam around my ears, and went into the water. Without effort I swam around the side of the bank.
>
> The water was very cold, but I had been reading a book about the "etheric double" and was inspired by the thought that, when you have perfected your body and lead a pure life, you are able to use your second body to communicate with the living spirits of nature: the little elves and fairies who evidently do exist at some stage of awareness.
>
> So, as I swam, my strokes long and sleek, the shadows of the rocks coming out from underneath the water like sunken civilization, the slight wind and clouds bringing me energy, I evoked just to my left the spirit of the lake to swim with me. And I started to imagine that there were streamers of warm energy going through the very marrow of my bones as the icy water started to finger its way into my joints and muscles.
>
> I found there was a seven- to eight-degree difference of temperature if I swam close to shore rather than out where it was very deep. The coldness and numbness made me forget my body for periods of time. I sent my consciousness to Jeanne in the house, knowing, she was trying to work on the proposal with Chuck and the children cluttering the environment. As I pulled my strokes, kicked my feet, and breathed, I turned my head just enough to watch out for motorboats.
>
> One came a bit too close. Then, in the middle of the lake, a canoe came by and a woman said, "Good, God, what are you doing, lady?" And the

man with her tried to put me down, "Don't you know better?" This was a precious swim and I was using all the concentration I could muster to stay warm and visualize myself swimming with the little elves and fairies. I didn't want these people in my conciousness, so I evoked a protective shield and felt myself being surrounded by a warm womb as I continued, stroke after stroke. My eyes were opened to the clear, pure water, and I gazed down at the ledges and rocks, and purple, black, and blue water beneath me.

I soon made the other side and got up on the rock. I wanted to lie in the sun, but knew I would chill off. Indeed, it was quite a long way. So I quickly checked out my body and realized it had not been nearly as difficult as I had thought it would be. I dove into the water and started back. Halfway across the lake, Jeanne came out after me in a sailboat. "Dyveke, there are more motorboats on the lake. I was getting worried about you and I really didn't think you could swim back." I laughed, and said, "That's all right, Jeanne. Go on and take the boat back and let me swim." So I swam a bit more. Finally I did get into the boat, having swum for perhaps two hours.

Later I reflected on the little channel and the trees, the vistas in all directions, the spirit of the lake in my psyche, the joy in attempting all kinds of visualizations to play the edges of my own capacity for endurance and centeredness. It was like a musical composition in ice water. I didn't do it to prove anything. I did it because I wanted an artistic moment alone with myself to appreciate that which I had sculpted — my flesh vehicle — and to explore the realms of my own consciousness.

And so I swam with the spirit of the lake and the little fairies of the water, and I sent my consciousness to Jeanne. I got into a rhythm and music came to me. I looked at the vast depths of the water and my body stroked and kicked. The rocks, the trees, the clouds all sent streamers of energy and I felt alive and vital and appreciative of the life force, the prana force, all about me. I thought of many things I must do to perfect my cellular system to become a vibrating echo of the lake.

Prelude to
Nutritional Awareness
for Energy and Health

It seems important at the outset to state my opinion about writing a chapter on nutrition in a book on Lifestyle Training. I could write an entire book on nutrition, shopping, reading labels, eating, my personal biases. I do not didactically advocate one diet for everyone but offer, rather, several options depending on your individual needs. There are some basic rules and "no no's" and at the end of the chapter I will outline *one* of the finest basic diets I know for some people, especially *athletes in training*. However, it is important to see this recommendation in the context of the ideas of the chapter. I want to expose and expand your awareness about your nutrition and give you flexible guidelines so that you can become your own best monitor and coach.

At its best, what you eat can give you tremendous energy and well as protect you from degenerative diseases such as arteriosclerosis, high blood pressure, and diabetes. It can also help your body build its resistance to infectious diseases. If a degenerative disease is already operating in your body, the food you eat can help to arrest and sometimes reverse the disease. At its worst, what you eat can bring about and accelerate degenerative diseases and, equally bad, rob you of the energy that is rightfully yours.

You will have energy when you are on a diet that is right for you. But finding this diet may not be simple. John's story is a good example of how an otherwise healthy person can eat what would generally be an excellent diet, but which for him was pure poison.

> For some months, I had been concerned with my diet. I had started a running program and was really feeling good. But at the same time I knew from my cursory reading that I had some gaps in my own nutrition and was eating some questionable foods. Also I was in a period of con-

113

stant stress in my job. The more I read about nutrition, the more confused I became. One physician friend told me of the horrors of drinking milk, which I had done all my life. I tried to stop drinking milk. Then another physician friend said that milk was a perfect food. I started drinking it again. A therapist told me that I should be taking B vitamins for stress as well as A and C and minerals. My personal physician told me that vitamins were a waste of my money. He also told me that I should cut down on red meat. Another doctor told me to cut out *all* meat.

Deep down inside, I wanted to find a book that would lay it all out for me; tell me exactly what to do and why. I would certainly follow such instructions if I could find them. Then I read Donald Ardell's *High Level Wellness*. He said, in effect, that the solution I was looking for did not exist, that I would have to take personal responsibility for my own nutrition, and that I would have to go through a long process to discover what was right for me. My experience convinced me that he was right, so I plunged in for more reading and experimentation.

Finally I found what I believe is a key book on the subject of nutrition, *Live Longer Now* by J. Leonard, J.L. Hofer, and N. Pritikin. The book makes the point that there are good carbohydrates, the starches, and bad carbohydrates, the simple sugars. The authors also show from the analysis of many research studies that a diet high in complex carbohydrates, with moderate protein and almost no fat, can prevent degenerative disease and, for those who are already afflicted, help reverse it. They paint a graphic picture of what happens in the arteries when plaques form and begin to clog them. They also point out what can happen when a piece breaks off and rushes down an artery.

To me, the argument was so strong that I determined to begin a high-carbohydrate, low-fat diet immediately. If I had arterial damage, I could begin to reverse it. If not, I would keep it from happening.

The book gives five commandments:

1. Don't eat fats or oils.
2. Don't eat sugar.
3. Don't eat salt.
4. Don't eat cholesterol.
5. Don't drink coffee or tea.

I had never used coffee or tea and I had kept my sugar intake pretty low. A few months ago I had cut out the last of the soft drinks. Now I began to carefully inspect food labels to be sure that no sugar was slipping in without my being aware of it. Whenever I saw sugar, dextrose, sucrose, corn or maple syrup, honey, brown sugar, I rejected the item. I had always thought an active person needed extra salt, but I stopped putting it in when I prepared my oatmeal. I also stopped putting any salt on my other foods. I stopped eating potato chips. I still ate some popcorn with salt and Triscuits, which are liberally salted. I had been back and forth on eggs and this book persuaded me to drop them completely, as well as shellfish and animal organs. This would help me with the cholesterol problem.

This left the number 1 commandment, fats. I began to make a conscious attempt to exclude fats from my diet. I wasn't using much milk, but I changed from whole to low-fat. I stopped having salad dressing on my sandwiches. I stopped eating tuna packed in oil because of the high fat content.

I knew what to expect. Simple carbohydrates lead the digestive system to dump sugar very quickly into the bloodstream and cause an oversupply of insulin. This results in a drop in blood sugar. By cutting out simple carbohydrates, I could avoid the headaches, depression, lack of energy, and anxiety that accompany this hypoglocemic-like state. Complex carbohydrates work differently. They are converted by the digestive system into simple sugars, but are diffused very slowly into the bloodstream, thereby keeping the blood sugar stable. By eating lots of complex carbohydrates, I could keep a steady stream of energy going to my body.

Thus I put a high-carbohydrate diet together. During a typical day, I would eat

1. Four servings of oatmeal with two bananas, yogurt, and low fat milk.
2. Two banana sandwiches on wholewheat bread with no salad dressing.
3. Two tomato sandwiches on wholewheat bread with no salad dressing.
4. Four oranges.
5. A large slice of watermelon.
6. A bowl of grapenuts with skim milk and yogurt.
7. Several times a week, I'd have a large plate of spaghetti.

While this was certainly not a perfect example of the diet in *Live Longer Now*, it was certainly high in complex carbohydrates. Of the items in the diet, I mentioned, only the yogurt is not on the accepted food list.

But what happened to me was almost beyond my belief. First, though I had two regular bowel movements a day, I had a terrible problem with gas. Second, and worse, I had absolutely no energy. I had wanted to start a strength-training program and had bought a portable, easy-to-use device. But I literally couldn't bear to think of trying it. My mind just blocked completely.

I was in the midst of a flexibility program that involved doing about 30 minutes of yoga stretches a day. I just didn't seem to have the energy to do them. When I was able to convince myself to try, I'd be exhausted after finishing, even if I did them when I first got up. I had been a little lax about my running. When I tried to resume it, I had a hard time completing a trail that I used to manage easily. But worse, I'd have to take a nap when I got back home.

Third, sometimes I'd feel energetic. Then I'd eat and immediately feel as though I couldn't face life until I had a nap. I'd feel absolutely exhausted. My mind was *cloudy*. I'd sleep for three hours, wake up and eat and then be exhausted again. And this on top of ten hours of sleep the night before. At first I attributed these effects to the jet lag from a west coast trip I had just taken. Then, when it didn't clear up, I thought it was tension from a business deal that I was trying to complete. But even when I resolved the deal in a favorable way, I was still exhausted. And the exhaustion continued. I had heard a lot about carbohydrate loading for athletes. Why wasn't the high carbohydrate diet working for me?

About this time I picked up another popular book on nutrition and to my utter horror read the author's conclusion that a high-protein, low-carbohydrate diet was the answer to many people's energy problems. I didn't want to believe this because of the strong, well-documented work on the high-carbohydrate diet. Nevertheless, I started a tentative swing toward protein. Being attuned to nutritional labels, I was immediately able to spot cottage cheese as being high in protein. Lima beans also looked promising.

About a month prior to this I had met a former pharmacist, now biochemist, Dr. Steve Bajon, founder of Dynamic Nutrition Analysis in San Diego. Steve had taken a hair sample from me and sent it to a laboratory to determine my mineral balance. Steve had said, "There is no such thing as one optimal diet for everyone. Because of the differences in soil conditions, an individual's reactions to food in the form of allergies, his past eating habits, each person's diet needs to be somewhat different. One person's meat is another person's poison."

Suddenly, in the midst of my own personal energy crisis, the results of my hair sample came back. Steve said, "You are a high metabolizer. You need protein. You should limit your carbohydrates. You have a calcium, iron, and zinc deficiency and a sodium and potassium overload. You should avoid wheat."

I immediately added milk, eggs and sources high in protein to my diet. On a typical day I would eat:

1. Three soft-boiled eggs.
2. Two servings of cottage cheese
3. A can of water-packed tuna with 70 gram of proteins.
4. A can of lima beans.
5. Six cups of whole milk.
6. A tomato.
7. A bowl of oatmeal with yogurt.
8. Two peaches or apples.

Immediately my energy level shot up. From the second day, my requirement for sleep went down. I was much more alive during the whole work day and had really high energy at night. The feeling of not being able to face problems disappeared. I felt like pursuing my hobbies, going out, resuming my stretching and running, and beginning my strength training.

And all of this happened before I got Steve's package of therapeutic vitamin and mineral supplements. Within two weeks of beginning the supplements, I noticed that my energy was high and constant throughout the day and into the evening. The burning sensation I used to notice in my eyes when I had to work in the evenings, disappeared. I felt like a completely new person. This feeling has lasted for many months and shows no sign of going away.

Chapter Six:
Nutritional Awareness
for Energy and Health

There is a powerful lesson in John's experience described in the prelude to this chapter. First, it is a good example of the pitfalls that face people who try to clean up their nutrition. There are so many contradictory opinions from people who qualify as experts that it is hard for a layperson to arrive at a solution.

Second, John's experience illustrates how crucial it is to realize that we are all individuals, and what works for one may not work for another. Many people have benefited from the high complex carbohydrate diet recommended in *Live Longer Now*. I consider it one of the landmark books on nutrition. But this diet didn't work for John. The Pritiken diet is strictly a therapeutic diet, very deficient in many important nutrients and cannot be used by anyone except those with cardiovascular disorders. It is too low in fats and fat-soluable vitamins. If he had continued a high complex carbohydrate diet of the type he had started, he could have done great damage to himself.

Third, John's experience points up how important nutrition is in setting up a Lifestyle Training Program. A diet that provides the wrong fuel to the body can stop a Lifestyle Training Program cold. John's program literally came to a halt when he went on a diet that was inappropriate for him. He thought that it was psychological, that he didn't have enough will power. But his diet had totally debilitated his will. It returned as strong as ever when he got on an appropriate diet.

Imagine how hard it would be to start a Lifestyle Training Program feeling like John. I believe that you can avoid many problems of motivation in your training program by first taking care of your nutrition. In fact, it may be impractical to start a program until you do deal with your nutrition. John, who knew all the theory and benefits of a training program, was unable to keep his program going when he was on the wrong nutritional track.

In this chapter, I am not going to advocate specific diets such as high protein or high carbohydrate. Rather I want to help you develop a deeper level of awareness concerning nutrition and give you some practical tools for finding your optimal diet. I want you to adopt a whole new attitude toward food. *Begin to see foods in terms of the fuel they provide your body, not in terms of the psychological satisfaction they give you.* Begin to visualize what happens inside your body when you take in certain nutrients. Be willing to experiment a little in order to find what suits your needs. I will tell you about the Hair Sample Analysis, a technique that can unambiguously reveal what vitamin and mineral supplements you need.

Such an approach can help you make a more meaningful evaluation of the nutritional advice with which you are constantly bombarded. You will begin to make a more informed choice about the foods you allow inside your body. You will no longer choose foods just because some authority says they are good for you.

Developing Nutritional Awareness

In this section, I want to give you some basic tools that can help you begin to make some of the important decisions about your own nutrition. As the body functions from day to day, we can either expedite these functions by providing the type of fuel the body needs, or we can impede them by giving the body the wrong fuel mixture. There is a very good analogy here with cars. Some cars run better on premium gasoline, some on regular, some on unleaded. If you use the gasoline your car was constructed to use, then it is has the potential for the performance it is supposed to give. If you put in the wrong kind of gasoline, you will get a degradation of performance no matter what the state of the other components.

Your attempt to develop endurance, strength, flexibility, and the powers of the mind will be seriously impeded if your nutrition does not provide your body with the correct amounts of the nutrients it needs. You have seen in John's case how use of inappropriate fuel can bring a Lifestyle Training Program to a screeching halt. I can't tell you what your optimal diet should be, but I can help you begin to examine the subject with a new awareness.

The body needs five basic classes of nutrients in certain quantities in order to operate in an optimal fashion. And different bodies need different proportions of these nutrients. The five nutrients are proteins, carbohydrates, fats, vitamins and minerals. We were all taught this in school. But for many of us, it didn't mean too much at the time. We had a lot of energy then. But now, if you are tired a lot, if you suffer from general anxiety, if your ambition and motivation have all but disappeared, if you have tension headaches, sore muscles, if you just don't feel good in general, the culprit could be your nutrition. And to eliminate these problems, you need to be more aware of what foods you are putting in your body.

Nutritional Labels

When you go into a grocery store and walk down the aisles, you have certain reactions to certain foods. You see an apple as that thing you love to bite into when you've been out working in the garden, that piece of food you used to pull off your grandfather's tree when you were young. A soft drink is something you used to grab after your baseball team won a tough game. When you are in a restaurant, the same thing happens. You see fried chicken on the menu and immediately remember how mother used to cook it on Sunday. You'd sit around the table with your brothers and sisters, aunts, uncles, and cousins, and laugh, talk, and eat fried chicken.

These reactions are based on learned responses to certain foods. So when we see a soft drink, we don't think about about simple carbohydrates, caffeine, and a whole series of foreign chemicals that our body doesn't need or want. We think about "the pause that refreshes." When we see fried chicken, we don't think about protein and fat and unwanted hormones; we think about joy and family closeness, about mother's love. We have unpleasant reactions to some foods, based not on nutritional value but on some unpleasant happening in the past. "We ate nothing but lima beans when we first got married because that was all we could afford. I never want to see another lima bean."

These psychological reactions have their place in our lives, but when we are concerned with trying to feel good, to have energy and motivation, we have to consider the fuel we are putting into our bodies in another light. We have to begin to pay attention to what nutrients and nonnutrients are in the food we eat. Start to see a soft drink as carbonated water, sugar, artificial flavors, artificial colors, caffine, stannous chloride, high calories. See a one pound t-bone steak as 1,596 calories with 59 grams of protein and 150 grams of fat.

Step one is to develop a new way of seeing food. In order to practice this new awareness, you must get familiar with the composition of foods. You can begin with the nutritional information on many cans, boxes, bottles, and bags. The nutritional information generally tells you what nutrients are in a given serving size. The proteins, carbohydrates, and fat are given in grams, and the vitamins and minerals in the percentage of U.S. Recommended Daily Allowance (U.S. RDA). Many nutritionists disagree on the recommendations. The vitamin C recommendation may be large enough to keep you from getting scurvy, but not to ward off excessive fatigue. But these RDAs are a starting point to get you acquainted with what you are putting into your body.

Then there is the *list of the ingredients* in order of amount, from largest to smallest. This list is very important, since you could have two foods with the same number of calories, grams of protein, carbohydrates, and fat, but nutrients in the two foods could be coming from quite different ingredients. For example, very few labels distinguish between simple and complex carbohydrates, but the effect of these two types on the body is dramatically different, as we will see later in this chapter.

One of the most instructive examples I have found of nutritional labels is that on Kellogg's All-Bran, shown in Table One.

This is a lot of information, and it is printed in pretty small type on the All-Bran box. But with a little practice you can spend just a few seconds with a nutritional label and make a quick decision as to whether you want those things going into your body and into the bodies of your family. For example, a person allergic to wheat can see that All-Bran is not for them. And for people who want to minimize the amount of sugar going into their body, All-Bran will not be acceptable since the list of ingredients tells us the sugar in this product is second in amount only to the wheat bran.

One of the main reasons for eating this cereal is to add roughage to the diet to aid in elimination. And this cereal certainly has roughage, two grams of non-nutritive crude fiber per serving. But I might point out that this same fiber can be gotten from bran itself, avoiding the sugar and preservatives found here. By studying the label, you can tell something about the compromises you will be making if you use this product.

A person who is on a high-protein, low-carbohydrate diet can immediately see that this product does not fit very well into that diet. There is barely any protein. The cereal is mostly carbohydrates. So this person might have to decide between the beneficial effects of the crude fiber and the high carbohydrate content. Even a person on a high-carbohydrate diet would have pause for reflection since the carbohydrate analysis shows that six grams of the carbohydrates are in the form of simple carbohydrates (simple sucrose and other dietary fiber). (In most labels the carbohydrate information is not broken down this way. When this information is not explicitly stated, the word *sugar* in the list of ingredients is a tipoff that you'd better pay special attention to the carbohydrates.)

The list of ingredients also shows what vitamins and minerals have been added. These can be checked against the percentages of vitamins to determine which are inherent in the product and which have been added. In All-Bran, the zinc was added but not the iron.

Now compare the All-Bran with Quick Quaker Oats in Table Two.

This label has several points of interest. First, nothing is added. The ingredients list only contains one item, rolled oats. Second, there are two addi-

Table One
Kellogg's All-Bran, fortified with ten essential vitamins and minerals

Serving Size	1 oz (= 1/3 cup)	With 1/2 cup whole milk	1/2 cup whole milk alone
Servings/Container	16		
Calories	70	150	80
Protein	3 gm	7 gm	4
Carbohydrates	22 gm	28 gm	6
Fat	1 gm	5 gm	4

Carbohydrate information:

Starch and related carbohydrates	8 gm	8 gm	0
Sucrose and other sugars	6 gm	12 gm	6
Dietary fiber	8 gm	8 gm	0
Total carbohydrates	22 gm	28 gm	6

Contains 8 gm dietary fiber, including 2 gm (7.5%) by weight), non-nutritive crude fiber.

Percentage of U.S. Recommended Daily Allowance (U.S. RDA)

Protein	4	15	11
Vitamin A	25	30	5
Vitamin C	25	25	0
Thiamine B1	25	30	5
Riboflavin B2	25	35	10
Niacin	25	25	0
Calcium	2	15	13
Iron	25	25	0
Vitamin D	10	25	15
Vitamin B6	25	25	0
Folic Acid	25	25	0
Phosphorus	25	35	10
Magnesium	25	30	5
Zinc	25	30	5
Copper	15	15	0

Ingredients

Wheat Bran
Sugar
Salt
Malt flavoring
Sodium ascorbate (C)
Vitamin A palmitate
Reduced iron
Zinc oxide

Ascorbic acid (C)
Pyridoxine hydrochloride (B6)
Thiamin hydrochloride (B1)
Riboflavin (B2)
Niacinamide
Folic acid
Vitamin D2

Ingredient Analysis

Wheat bran
Sugar
Malt flavoring
Salt

Table Two
Quick Quaker Oats

Serving Size	1 oz (= 1/3 cup)	With 1/2 cup whole milk	1/2 cup whole milk alone
Servings/Container	42		
Calories	110	190	80
Protein	5 gm	9 gm	4
Carbohydrates	18 gm	24 gm	6
Fat	2 gm	6 gm	4

.3 gm fiber per serving

Cholesterol	0	15 mg	15 mg
Sodium	10 mg	15 mg	5 mg

Percentage of U.S. Recommended Daily Allowance (U.S. RDA)

Protein	15	15	0
Vitamin A	†	2	2
Vitamin C	†	†	0
Thiamine B1	10	10	0
Riboflavin B2	†	10	10
Niacin	†	†	0
Calcium	†	10	10
Iron	4	4	0
Vitamin D	†	10	10
Phosphorus	8	20	12

†Contains less than 2% of the U.S. RDA of these nutrients.

Ingredients

100% rolled oats

tional categories listed here: the amount of cholesterol and the amount of sodium. But note that the sodium content here does not include the salt recommended in preparing the cereal. While it can be cooked without the salt, most people automatically add it because it is in the cooking instructions. This, of course, alters the sodium content. As compared to the All-Bran, the Oats look rather skimpy in terms of vitamins and minerals. They are lower in carbohydrates, 18 as opposed to 22; and most likely the difference is due to the lack of simple carbohydrates. But if a person adds sugar to the oatmeal, the carbohydrates are going to go up, and from the wrong direction, simple rather than complex. The number of calories is also quite different: 110 for the oats, 70 for the bran.

Also notice the difference in vitamins and mineral attributed to the whole milk from the two labels. There is a difference both in amount and presence. If you get a carton of whole milk and look at its nutritional information, you'll probably see even more difference. The bran label shows vitamin A as 5%; whereas for the oats, it is shown as 2%. Neither magnesium nor zinc is shown on the oats label.

As far as commercial cereals are concerned, this is probably one of the most acceptable. However, we should always be aware that it is possible to buy completely natural, unprocessed cereals and grains with nothing artificial added.

Now look at the nutritional label for a carton of whole milk in Table Three.

You can see from the nutrients attributed to milk on the two cereals versus an actual label from milk that, if you're trying to find out what is actually going into your body, you need to look at the label on that product, not at what some other source may have implied. Notice that nothing is said in the milk label about sodium or cholesterol content. We have the Oats label to thank for calling this possibility to our attention.

A useful exercise as you begin to develop awareness in the nutritional content of food is to go to your local supermarket or grocery store and study the labels on various products.

Peanut butter is an item in which the fat content outstrips both the protein and carbohydrate content. Tuna packed in water is extremely high in protein, with almost no carbohydrate and moderate fat. But compare tuna packed in water with tuna packed in oil and look at the fat content of the latter. Another interesting comparison is Del Monte Green Lima Beans and Del Monte French Style Green Beans. Among other things, you will see that it takes four servings of the green beans to give you the approximate nutritional equalivant of one serving of lima beans.

As part of your awareness training, I recommend *Composition of Foods* by B. K. Watt and A. L. Merrill, a 190-page book showing the caloric, protein, carbohydrate, fat, vitamin, and mineral content of thousands of foods. You can use this to get information on foods that don't yet have nutritional labels, and to make comparisons between various types of food.

I also strongly recommend the Nutrition Slide Guide available for $3.00 from Dunn & Reidman, Box 241, Pacific Palisades, CA 90272. This is a cardboard device that lets you instantly determine the nutritional content of 321 different foods. You can determine in seconds, for each food listed, the same type of nutritional information that you find on food packages. It is compact and fits easily into a purse or briefcase.

With this background, you are now ready to begin practicing a new awareness toward food. Go into a grocery store and choose a food. Relax and see what comes to your mind when you see the food. What associations does it have from your past? Do you like it? Does it taste good? Is it reasonably priced? Now let these associations fade away and pick up the food. Study the ingredients on the nutritional label. Now, in your mind, see this particular food in terms of its nutritional content. See it as the individual ingredients listed on the label. For example, see a loaf of bread as ground

Table Three
West Lynn Creamery Homogenized Vitamin D Milk

Serving Size	1 cup, half pint
Servings/Container	1
Calories	150
Protein	8 gm
Carbohydrates	11 gm
Fat	8 gm

Percentage of U.S. Recommended Daily Allowance (U.S. RDA)

Protein	20
Vitamin A	4
Vitamin C	4
Thiamine B1	6
Riboflavin B2	25
Niacin	†
Calcium	30
Iron	†
Vitamin D	25
Vitamin B6	4
Vitamin B12	15
Phosphorus	20
Magnesium	8
Zinc	4
Pantothenic Acid	6

†Contains less than 2% of the U.S. RDA of these nutrients.

Ingredients

Milk, Vitamin D3 added

flour, water, nonfat milk, unsulphured molasses, vegetable shortening, corn syrup, yeast, salt, etc. Realize that you're getting all these things when you eat the bread.

Now look at the nutritional content and visualize two slices of the bread. See them as 4 grams of protein, 23 grams of carbohydrate, 2 grams of fat, with vitamins B1, B2, niacin, calcium, and iron. Stay with this image. Whenever you see bread in the future, be aware of it as potential fuel for your body.

Once you have determined what your body needs, you can then determine how a particular food rates as fuel for your body. Until you are really satisfied with your nutrition, begin to see foods as their nutritional content.

My main purpose here is to help you become more discriminate in choosing the food you eat. You must begin to change your criteria for choice. It can no longer be based on what you learned to eat when you were growing, what likes and dislikes you have learned as you've gone out on your own, the price tag on the item, etc. Too often people assume that if you can buy it in a reputable store, it must be all right. This makes no more sense than the other often-held belief that something printed in a book, magazine, or newspaper must be true. You probably long ago realized the foolishness of the latter, but what about the former? How you feel, how your body functions, the clarity of your mind, all depend on what you eat. It's time to make the connection between lack of energy, muscle aches, anxiety, and the fuel you are providing your body.

One of the unfortunate aspects of the human potential movement is that it sometimes gets divided into camps. There are some who see the mind as the key to all our problems. Learn to relax and make positive suggestions to yourself and you can get the energy you need. Others say that it is all a matter of physical training. Do enough running, swimming, and stretching, and you'll have all the energy you could ever ask for. Then there are those who say that good nutrition is sufficient. But it is becoming more and more clear that we must take care of nutrition, physical training, *and* our minds in order to have a smoothly functioning organism.

Some people point out that going on a physical training program often creates a desire to clean up nutrition. But this is approaching the matter the hard way. And, for many people, the old nutrition will provide such a drag that a program will never be started. Contrast knowing about the correct fuel for your car and getting the engine tuned up with choosing to get your exercise tuned up while waiting till later to change to the proper fuel.

It is clear that nutrition is the starting point on the path to optimal health, just as the gasoline we put in our cars is the starting point for a smoothly running car. Cars won't run without gasoline and won't run well without the right kind of gasoline. Our bodies won't run without fuel and won't run well, no matter what else we do, without the right kind of fuel. We need to give our cars periodic tune-ups, get new tires, have the wheels balanced. But if we're using regular gas in a car that needs premium, none of the other things is going to give us optimal performance.

What Happens to the Food We Eat

The second step in the process of developing nutritional awareness is to learn what happens to the food we eat. We must begin to connect our eating with what happens in our bodies when we eat a certain food. We have all become too accustomed to the psychological aspects of eating as they relate to how the food tastes, where we're eating, who we're eating with. Our likes and dislikes of certain foods are largely a learned function. And they can be modified.

One of the big problems is that we not only want our hunger satisfied, we want it satisfied with certain foods. And while these foods may temporarily satisfy us psychologically, they are not necessarily good for us physically. *And*, in the long run, they may cause us psychological harm.

The purpose of trying to bring about good nutrition is not to make life more bleak and dull by having to eat bland food. Good nutrition needn't take away from the beauty of an eating experience; a nice restaurant with soft lights, music, friends. Good nutrition needn't involve the termination of such experiences. But it certainly may involve changing some of the things we order when we are in those situations. And it may even involve deleting some items from our diet that we like, indeed love.

But if the whole process is approached with awareness, it will happen rather naturally. To develop this new awareness you need to get firmly in mind a general model of what happens to the food you eat. Once you have this basic model in mind, review it just prior to eating. Then start to expand this general model to include the more specific things that happen when a given nutrient is involved.

Suppose you eat a meal that includes proteins, carbohydrates, fats, vitamins, minerals, and some fiber such as cellulose or bran that your body cannot digest. The digestive system breaks the food down into the basic components: glucose, amino acids, fatty acid, and glycerol. The process begins in the stomach where the food is reduced to pulp. After about an hour the pulp goes to the small intestine where the pancreas and gall bladder supply digestive juices that convert complex carbohydrates into glucose, protein into amino acids, and fats into fatty acid and glycerol.

The amino acids and glucose go into the blood capillaries after they are broken down. Simple carbohydrates are broken down very quickly and dumped into the bloodstream. The fatty acids and glycerol go to the liver where fats are synthesized and minerals and vitamins are stored. Roughage, which can't be digested by the body, helps the food move through the digestive system and is then passed with other wastes to the large intestine.

At the end of the digestive process, the nutrients are deposited into the blood along with oxygen from the lungs. The nutrients and oxygen are carried through the arteries to the body's cells to be used in building and repairing cells and providing us with energy. Carbon dioxide and other wastes are returned through the veins to various parts of the body for elimination.

It is important to recognize that specific things are being done with any food you take into your body and that these things have a specific effect on how you function and how you feel both physically and psychologically.

About half of the body's energy comes from starch and sugar (complex and simple carbohydrates) and the other half from protein and fat. Unneeded carbohydrates are stored in the body in a form called glycogen. If you failed to replenish the supply of carbohydrates in your body for a while, there would be enough stored glycogen to last for two days. Then the body would start calling on the stored fats, triglyceride.

Vitamins and minerals are needed to help metabolize the food you eat. The best definition I've seen of vitamins and minerals comes from *Live Longer Now*:

> A vitamin is
> 1. An organic chemical.
> 2. It is present in foods in extremely small amounts.
> 3. It is essential for normal health.
> 4. A specific disease occurs if it is absent.
> 5. It cannot be made by the body.
>
> Minerals follow this same definition except that they are inorganic chemicals. A hormone is the same as a vitamin except that the body can make it by itself. (Page 102)

Vitamins and minerals are important. For instance, it is easy to see why proper vitamin intake can markedly affect athletic performance. Vitamin A keeps connective tissues young and aids tissue oxygenation. It affects sex hormone metabolism which in turn affects the adrenals, which are central to the stress system. The B-complex vitamins reduce glucose and metabolism of carbohydrates and affect endurance, circulation, and red blood count. B6 helps protein and fat metabolism and aids in producing antibodies. B12 regenerates red blood cells and aids the healing processes. Vitamin C strengthens connective tissue and is necessary for the adrenal and thyroid glands to function. Vitamin C protects aginst stress and is a powerful detoxicant. Vitamin E improves circulation and oxygenation of the tissues.

A deficiency in a given vitamin or mineral can cause a specific disease. For example, a vitamin A deficiency can cause night blindness; vitamin D, rickets; vitamin C, scurvy; niacin, pellagra. In the case of minerals, a calcium deficiency can cause bone disease; magnesium, growth retardation; iron, anemia. But a vitamin or mineral can have more than one use. Vitamins and minerals in certain doses have cleared up insomnia, leg cramps, arthritis, depression, anxiety, headaches, fatigue.

Excessive dosages of certain vitamins and minerals can cause problems. There are water-soluble vitamins, C and the Bs, and fat-soluble vitamins, A, D, E and K. The fat-soluble vitamins can be accumulated in the body and therefore overdosage can be a problem. It can also be a problem with minerals. So we must learn to use discrimination with regard to vitamins and minerals. Indiscriminate use can cause serious problems. And as Dr. Robert Atkins points out in *Superenergy Diet*:

> Vitamins, even when they are desperately needed, when used without the proper diet, rarely produce much tangible benefit.

Make an attempt every time you eat anything, whether a full meal or a snack, to briefly review what will happen to the food. It will be broken down into the nutrients and non-nutrients it contains, and sent to the cells for immediate use, stored for later use, or eliminated from the body.

What Happens with Specific Nutrients

Once you have in mind the general model of what happens to the food you eat, it will be very helpful to get a model of what happens with individual nutrients. The most important of these specific models is that for carbohydrates.

Carbohydrates can be divided into three distinct types: cellulose, simple carbohydrates, and complex carbohydrates. Cellulose can't be used by the body as a nutrient, but it *is* used to help move food through the digestive system and contribute to good elimination. Simple carbohydrates, such as table sugar, some fruits, the lactose in milk, are composed of two sugar molecules. Complex carbohydrates, such as lima beans, are composed of thousands of sugar molecules. In the end, complex carbohydrates are broken up by the body into simple sugars. But the effect of eating food with simple carbohydrates versus food with complex carbohydrates is dramatically different.

Simple Carbohydrates: Putting Out the Fire

We spend 4 billion dollars a year on candy bars, 3 billion on soft drinks, and 11.5 billion on alcohol (*The Complete Runner*, Runner's World, pg. 132).

There is a direct relationship between people who get hooked on sugar as children and who get hooked on alcohol as adults.

Suppose you drink a soft drink, eat a piece of cake, or some cookies. All of these items contain mainly simple carbohydrates. This means that the body can immediately break the carbohydrates down into simple sugars and put them directly into the blood. In your visualization, picture your system getting a severe jolt as the sugar is dumped into your blood. See this in your mind's eye as a fire, a blazing fire in your bloodstream. There is a feeling of high energy in your body for a while. Then see your pancreas suddenly called into action to produce the insulin needed to metabolize the sudden influx of sugar.

Picture the process of pancreas response as a fire station answering a three-alarm fire. There is an emergency. The fire fighters dump tons of water on the burning building. Finally the fire is extinguished and the site of the fire is a soggy mess. This is like the reaction of the pancreas as it produces insulin. It produces so much that your are actually left with too little sugar in your blood, low blood sugar, and there is a feeling of low energy and depression.

This is what happens every time you bombard your body with simple carbohydrates. To add insult to injury, the simple sugars raise the fat level in your blood and result in additional weight. And furthermore, foods high in simple carbohydrates often have none of the vitamin and mineral nutrients needed to metabolize the simple carbohydrates, so the body must take these nutrients from storage.

Realize that the implicit visualization you often have when eating sweets, the picture of warmth, love, friendship, and satisfaction, is at great variance with what is actually happening inside your body. What is happening is analogous to what happens when you are frightened and your body begins to marshall resources to put up a fight or to get away from the source of danger.

Thus, even if you feel right now that you can't immediately cut simple carbohydrates from your diet, every time you are about to take them in, let your mind go through the simple visualization above and weigh that against the fleeting psychological benefits that you are trying to achieve. You may decide in some instances that it isn't worth the upset to your system. You may decide to forego the simple carbohydrates, or substitute something that will lead to a more desirable result in your body.

Complex Carbohydrates: Time-Release Energy

Most of us have developed a negative attitude toward carbohydrates. What has given carbohydrates their bad image is just what we described above. But all carbohydrates are not alike. Simple carbohydrates are quite different from complex carbohydrates. The digestive system breaks down complex carbohydrates (starches) into simple sugars of the type we get if we eat simple carbohydrates. These sugars are absolutely essential for the body to function properly, but it is *how* this happens that makes all the difference.

When you think of eating a food with complex carbohydrates, such as lima beans, apples, bananas, visualize the body taking in the food. It starts to break down the complex molecular structure into simple sugars and to get the sugar into the blood stream. There is a lot of work going on. Picture a complex structure that has been built with tinker toys. It is now being taken apart. There are all sorts of connections to undo. Rods have to be eased out of the holes they were earlier pushed into. It takes a while.

And so with complex carbohydrates, the process of breaking down the molecules takes a while. As a result, the sugar is released in manageable amounts, the pancreas thus produces insulin at a leisurely rate, and the blood sugar remains at a stable level over a long period of time. As an extra benefit during the dismantling of the complex carbohydrate, nutrients such as calcium, phosphorous, vitamin A, iron, etc. are extracted from the food with complex carbohydrates. The same kind of time-release function we're so familiar with in medicines is happening here. And with complex carbohydrates, we are getting a relatively clean energy source, with none of the complex waste products that result from the processing of fats and proteins.

Some Sample Diets and Their Deficiencies

Table Four shows three typical diets for a child, a manual laborer, and an athlete. Spend some time in visualizing what happens in the body of each of these people with a given meal.

How do these diets rate in terms of the overall nutritional needs of a typical person in each category? What can the three people above do to improve their diets that will lead to a significant improvement in their nutrition and, as a result, in how they feel?

How to Determine Your Optimal Diet

Many books have been written advocating many nutritional approaches. You should read some of these books. But in the end, you must realize that we are each very different in terms of the fuel our bodies need. In this matter, the analogy with cars is not good. There are usually fuel pumps with three kinds of gas at a typical service station. Unfortunately, the same is not true of fuel for the human body. The choice of fuel is staggering.

One thing you can do is to experiment with yourself and try various diets. See what effect they have on your energy level and your state of mind. Of course, you need information from your physician on whether any specific approach is likely to be harmful for you. For example, if you have atherosclerosis, you should experiment only under the eyes of professionals.

Hair Sample Analysis: Your Personal Nutritional and Supplement Guide

If you don't want to take the time and effort to do your own experimentation — and it can take a considerable amount of both — there is an approach that can cut down on the time required to put together the optimal diet for you. This approach is called Hair Sample Analysis.

In this procedure, about two teaspoons of hair is cut from back of your head with stainless steel scissors. The hair sample is sent to a laboratory where it is thoroughly washed and then put through an analysis to determine the mineral content of your body during the three months prior to the sample. The professional who takes the sample then studies the results, which indicate not only the deficiency, adequacy, or excess of a particular

Table Four
Three typical menus for a child, a manual laborer and an athlete

A CHILD'S MENU

Breakfast	Lunch	Snack	Dinner	Snack
Bowl Sugar Cereal with milk	Hot Dog French Fries Milk	Potato Chips Soft Drink	Spaghetti Meat Sauce Potato Chips Soft Drink	Cookies Soft Drink

A MANUAL LABORER

Breakfast	Lunch	Snack	Dinner	Snack
Oatmeal with Milk Bacon and eggs White Bread and butter Coffee	Hamburgers French Fries Soft Drink Apple Pie	Soft Drink Potato Chips	Steak • French Fries Canned Peas White Rolls Cake Coffee	Lemon Pie Beer Potato Chips

ATHLETE

Breakfast	Lunch	Snack	Dinner	Snack
Oatmeal with Milk Granola and Banana Orange	2 banana sandwiches on brown bread 2 Peaches	Almonds Pumpkin seeds Apple Orange	2 Tomato sandwiches on brown Spaghetti with tomato sauce	Banana, yogurt, granola Orange

mineral in your body, but also the ratios of certain minerals. It will also identify the presence of any toxic minerals in your body.

A knowledgeable professional can take these laboratory results and recommend a therapeutic diet that includes vitamin and mineral supplements and homeopathic remedies (see Chapter 10 for a full definition) for the toxins. Once your body has stabilized, the therapist will recommend a maintenance diet. You can repeat the analysis from time to time in order to keep track of what is happening in your body.

To give you a concrete example, I'm going to relate the results of a recent hair sample analysis Dr. Steve Bajon did for me.

Hair Sample Analysis: My Case Study

I had tried various nutritional programs for several years, and the high-protein, low-carbohydrate approach was my basic method of trying to maintain high energy and a reasonable weight. Then I started to read books such as *Diet for a Small Planet* by Lappee, and Shelton's books on nutrition. These books and the experts in nutrition in the holistic health field in Mill Valley, California, all recommended the opposite: high carbohydrate, low protein, and little or no dairy. They advocated lots of seeds, grains, nuts, yogurt. Subsequently, I switched to Dr. Paavo Airola's Optimum Diet, which is outlined later in this chapter.

At the same time, I was attempting to withdraw from premarin and diuril which had been prescribed years earlier, and which I later learned kept my body in a state of water retention and dehydration simultaneously. I *knew* something was not right. With all my physical exercise, I was constantly battling too much weight. I tried Leonard's and Pritikin's recommendations of no salt, oils, white flour, alcohol, or cholesterol (eggs, etc.) and found an immediate drop of 10-15 pounds in two weeks, and, over the next eight or nine months, a resurgence of energy and vitality. I went into very intensive training, faithfully following the regimen in their book.

Shortly after this, I started traveling and teaching extensively, which necessitated eating in restaurants. It was impossible to get organic food and retain the discipline as I had done in Mill Valley. Then I had a serious injury to my hamstring. Following a double-day training on Mt. Tamalpais, I fell and caught my leg under a stick. Despite all my knowledge of the healing modalities, I, like any injured athlete, had to accept the inevitable and *rest*. For some this would not be so cataclysmic, but I had been running at least ten to 12 miles a day, teaching or coaching the other hours of the day, and was physically active most of the time. In short, my entire body chemistry was thrown *out of balance*. It was only following a Hair Sample Analysis that I could determine the proper diet for me, with the proper supplements to eliminate the aluminum and copper toxicity that had accumulated in my body.

According to the computerized print-out, I was unable to metabolize carbohydrates; my thyroid was low, magnesium outrageously out of balance (thrown out of my system by the diuril), and the premarin had created a high copper condition. All this caused personality characteristics of extreme emotionalism, mood swings. I also showed some hypoglycemia and was sternly recommended not to take any caffeine or sugars. I do not eat sugar if possible, but had been a *coffee nut* for 30 years. I was hard-pressed to drop this last addiction until I could see graphically with big red and black lines what it was doing to my body chemistry. Figure One shows this analysis.

Over this past summer I have been able to resume my intensive training. My hamstring is completely healed. I take a variety of minerals and supplements especially prescribed for my particular biochemistry. My diet is moderate protein, low carbohydrate with lots of fresh vegetables, some fruits, some eggs. I cannot eat cheese (which I adore) and have even given up licorice, which I used to *sneak*. This summer I put a package of licorice on the shelf, read the label (corn syrup, wheat flour, sugar, coconut oil, citric acid, artificial flavor, vinegar, artificial color, mono- and diglycerides [emulsifier derived from vegetable oil]) and repeated: "Dyveke, do you want all that junk in your body?" I cannot eat grains, seeds, and nuts because of the high oil content and my inability to metabolize carbohydrates. (After my biochemistry is stabilized and I am completely detoxified, I may test them out again.)

This summer I also had an applied kineseology examination, the testing of muscles in the body to find imbalances (see Chapter 10), and homeopathic diagnosis, along with a blood count. I am allergic to yellow dye, which is in yellow cheese, and of which I have eaten a great deal over the years. According to Dr. Bajon, I cannot eat oranges, apples, spinach, grapefruit (all which I also adore), because it causes water retention. Dr. Bajon informs me that it takes six to eight weeks to detoxify aluminum and copper with proper homeopathic remedies and proper nutrition. That time has now passed, and I can attest that I feel a stabilizing effect in my emotional state and overall functioning. I do not crave the foods I shouldn't eat anymore. An internal thermostat seems to be regulating my psychological attachments to food, and I have a master plan that is steering me with confidence.

It's hard not to be enthusiastic. I've struggled for so many years in such a haphazard way and made such terrible mistakes. I want to help you on your path. I think the hair sample analysis is one of the most important tools to short-cut the laborious search to find the right nutritional program for you. Your mineral/vitamin/chemical balance is unique. You may have cadmium, lead, aluminum, or copper toxicity which is throwing off or deflecting your body chemistry, no matter how well you are attempting to eat. The Hair Sample Analysis costs about $60 with a consultation. Supplements cost me $75 the first month, $50 the second. Continuing supplements of Vitamin E, C, B-complex, etc., will probably cost an on-going $20 to $25 per month. Although I have used myself as an illustrative example, most of my clients also get a hair sample analysis to chart the appropriate nutritional and detoxification program to facilitate their Lifestyle Training Program.

Your Body is a Bio-Chemical Plant

A research physicist and sports training expert, Chuck Richardson, co-led a six-week training program in the spring of 1976, titled "Higher Dimensions of Awareness through Physical Training." The following data were prepared for assistants I was training during a five-state conference titled "Women in Motion." We decided it was important to share the *basic scientific data* about body chemistry in order to lay the base for an understanding of the importance of proper nutrition.

Why nutrition? Your body is a fantastically complicated chemical plant. Everything it does involves chemicals. You have no solar cells, no atomic generators. Chemicals generate the electrical pulses you use to move, see, small, hear, think and even relax. Chemicals contract your muscles. At the same time they prevent you from tearing them to pieces by over-extending them. Chemicals generate the energy that heats, moves, and rebuilds your body.

Let me share some statistics:

In 1927 white bread was introduced into the United States. This bread is made from the endosperm of the wheat kernel. The endosperm contains most of the starch and a little of the protein that is in a wheat kernel. Left behind on the miller's floor is the bran or husk, which contains most of the vitamins and minerals, and most of the protein; along with the germ which contains all of the Vitamin E. If you plot the ever-increasing production for white bread alongside the ever-increasing incidence of heart disease in the U.S., you get two curves with startlingly similar slopes. When you tie this in with some of the successful research on Vitamin E in the treatment of heart disorders, it is alarming indeed. Sixteen million Americans are said to be suffering from heart diseases. Forty percent of the young men who were killed in Vietnam, on whom autopsies were per-formed, had signs of arteriosclerosis. We spend billions of dollars look-ing for a cure for heart disease when we know how to prevent most of it.

Why nutrition? Plot the consumption of white sugar in America over the last 50 years. Beside this curve, plot the incidence of dental cavities and gum disease. Their similarity is interesting. Today we have an estimated three million diabetics. Most of them, like most of the heart disease pa-tients, have a chemical problem. They do not have an infection or an in-jury. Insulin is a chemical, but it creates more problems than it solves.

Thirty million Americans suffer from arthritis. They have a chemical prob-lem. Most of them are told to take aspirin. Arthritis, headaches, upset stomachs do not occur because your body lacks aspirin. Your body can-not use aspirin in any form. It is a foreign substance and must be ex-pelled from the system. In other words, aspirins, create more problems for your body than the body already has. Every time you introduce a for-eign chemical into your plant, the plant must expend some of its re-sources to expel it. The body must expel the foreign substance at all costs, even to the loss of a vital organ. Alchohol is a foreign substance to the human body. It must be expelled even at the cost of a liver.

Red Dye No. 2 is a foreign substance to the body, yet it is found in virtual-ly all processed foods. When a child's body cannot expel this sub-stance, weird and terrible things happen. He may become so hyperac-tive that schools and parents resort to tranquilizers in order to control him. His problem is chemical and tranquilizers only add to the problem.

Four Commandments

1. Do not eat processed foods; hot dogs, sausage, cheeses, TV din-ners, salad dressings, ice cream, and hundreds of others. Processed foods contain so many dangerous chemicals it would take pages to list them. Ice cream, the soft, smooth stuff you buy in the supermarket, con-tains over 40 chemicals, none of which belongs in your body. These chemicals give ice cream that great appearance and long shelf life.

2. Do not eat sugar or sugar-coated products. Evidence is accumulating which indicates that sugar may be related to a number of diseases. You will get more sugar than you need from unsuspected sources anyway. Don't consume it directly.

3. Stop consuming poisonous chemicals that are found in coffee, cola drinks, deep-fried foods . . . to name a few. A breakfast of a cup of coffee, a doughnut, and a cigarette is a breakfast of poison.

4. Stop filling your system with no-value foods. You need all the capacity you have for valuable foods. Don't waste it on most dry cereals, instant rice, white bread. Their only contribution is calories, and we are the most over-caloried people on earth.

I cannot overemphasize the vast importance of an enlightened nutrition program. This self-education must assume top priority in your lifestyle reprogramming.

Don't Proselytize: Be an Example

As a person begins to deal with his or her nutrition, the concern tends to go beyond the individual. Often people become overbearing in their efforts to spread the word about a nutritional approach that has worked for them. This nearly always turns out to be a big mistake. The best course is usually to try to teach by presence. Get your nutrition together and be a sterling example. Bill took the right approach.

I started to work on my nutrition shortly after I was separated from my wife. At first, when I would see my kids we would joke about my new eating habits. I was heavily into grains, fruits, and vegetables. I'd take them to a fast food place and get a salad while they got hamburgers, french fries, and soft drinks. As I got more deeply into my nutritional changes, I began to feel a deep sense of guilt at what my family was eating. I realized that I had helped them establish their eating habits for the 20 years that I was with them. My wife had cooked the things that we liked, and as the children came along they mostly adapted to our tastes. I bought soft drinks in large quantities to save money. We ate out quite often, mostly at hamburger chains. We'd always buy lots of cookies, ice cream, etc., when we went shopping.

I really wanted my kids to change their nutritional habits. I cajoled them for a while. It just didn't work. Then I felt a lot of guilt. I keep saying to myself, "If I had just known what I know now, think of what their bodies would be like." But I've finally come to realize that all these regrets won't change anything. The best I can do now is to try to be a living example of what good nutrition can accomplish.

And this approach seems to be working. The kids know that I'm interested in nutrition. Now when they see things about nutrition on television and read about the subject in newspapers and magazines, they will ask my opinion. And they are gradually beginning to make some changes in their diet.

Dr. Paavo Airola's Optimum Diet

There are many authorities on good nutrition and I have found Dr. Paavo Airola's *Are You Confused?* and *How To Get Well* to be the most useful books. They list a good working menu for a nutritional way of life. Dr. Airola's books are excellent references and guidelines, and should be studied. The following is an excerpt from Dr. Airola's book *How To Get Well* (Published by Health Plus Publishers, P.O. Box 22001, Phoenix, Arizona 85028, $10.95.):

Here is the health-building and vitalizing Airola Diet, your health menu for a day:

Upon Arising

Glass of pure water, plain, or with freshly squeezed citrus juice: ½ lime, or ¼ lemon, or ½ grapefruit, or one orange to a glass of water.

OR: Large cup of warm herb tea sweetened with honey. Choice of rose hips, peppermint, camomile, or any of your favorite herbs.

OR: Glass of freshly made fruit juice from any available fruits or berries in season: apple, pineapple, orange, cherry, pear, etc. The juice should be diluted with water, half and half. No canned or frozen juices— the juice must be freshly made on you own juicer just before drinking, or squeezed from the fruit.

After this morning drink, you should walk for one hour in the fresh air, combining your walk with deep-breathing exercises and all the calisthenics you can manage to squeeze in. If you have a garden, or if you live on the farm, you should get in a couple of hours of hard physical labor.

Upon returning from your long walk, or garden work, and after a cold shower to wash the perspiration away, you are now, *but not before*, ready for your breakfast.

Breakfast

Fresh fruits: apple, orange, banana, grapes, grapefruit, or any available berries and fruits *in season*. All fruits preferably organically grown in your own locality and environment.

Cup of yogurt, kefir, or homemade soured milk, preferably goat's milk.

Handful of raw nuts, such as almonds, cashews, peanuts, or a couple of tablespoons of sunflower seeds, pumpkin seeds or sesame seeds. Nuts and seeds can be crushed or ground in your own seed grinder (sold in health food stores) and sprinkled over yogurt.

½ cup of homemade cottage cheese.

OR: Large bowl of fresh Fruit Salad à Là Airola.

OR: Bowl of rolled oats, uncooked, with 4-6 soaked prunes, or 2-3 figs, and a handful of unsulfured raisins.

Glass of raw, unpasteurized milk, preferably goat's milk, or yogurt.

OR: Bowl of sprouted wheat or other sprouted seeds with yogurt and/or available fresh fruits.

Midmorning Snack

One apple, banana, or other fruit.

Lunch

Bowl of whole-grain cereal, such as millet cereal, buckwheat cereal or Kruska. Any other available whole-grain cereals can be used such as oats, barley, rice, corn, etc. Dry milk powder (non-instant kind) can be added to the water when cereals are cooked.

Large glass of raw milk, preferably goat's milk.

One tablespoon of cold-pressed vegetable oil, and/or one tablespoon of honey can be used on cereal.

OR: Large bowl of fresh Fruit Salad à Là Airola (if not eaten for breakfast).

OR: Bowl of freshly prepared vegetable, pea or bean soup, or any other cooked vegetable dish, such as potatoes, squash, beans and corn tortillas, yams, etc. Kelp, sea salt, cold-pressed vegetable oil and fresh butter can be used for seasoning.

Glass of yogurt or other soured milk.

1-2 slices of whole-grain bread, preferably sourdough rye bread, 1 or 2 slices natural cheese, available at health food stores. Never use processed cheeses.

Midafternoon

Glass of fresh fruit or vegetable juice.

OR: Cup of your favorite herb tea, sweetened with honey.

OR: One apple, or other available fruit.

Dinner

Large bowl of fresh, green vegetable salad. Use any and all available vegetables, preferably those *in season*, including tomatoes, avocados and all available sprouts, such as alfalfa seed sprouts, mung bean sprouts, etc. Carrots, shredded red beets and onions should be staples with every salad. Garlic, if our social life permits. Salad should be attractively prepared and served with homemade dressing of lemon juice (or apple cider vinegar) and cold-pressed vegetable oil, seasoned with herbs, garlic powder, a little sea salt, cayenne pepper, etc. But all vegetables can be also placed attractively on the plate without mixing them into salad and eaten one at at time— this is, by far, the superior way of eating vegetables.

2 or 3 middle sized boiled or baked potatoes in jackets. Prepared cooked vegetable course, if desired: eggplant, artichoke, sweet potatoes, yams, squash or other vegetables. Use kelp powder or sea salt sparingly for seasoning, also any or all of the usual garden herbs.

Fresh homemade cottage cheese, or 1-2 slices of natural cheese.

Fresh butter or 1 tbsp. of cold-pressed vegetable oil (can be used on salad, soup or potatoes).

Glass of yogurt or other soured milk.

OR: Any of the recommended lunch choices, if fresh vegetable salad is eaten at lunch.

Bedtime Snack

Glass of fresh milk, or nut-milk, or seed-milk (made in electric liquifier from raw seeds or raw nuts and water and milk or without milk) with a tablespoon of honey.

OR: Glass of yogurt with brewer's yeast.

OR: Cup of your favorite herb tea with a slice of whole grain bread with butter and a slice of natural cheese.

OR: One apple.

Vital Points To Remember

1. The above menu is only a very general outline, a skeleton, around which an individual diet for optimum nutrition should be built. It can be followed as it is, of course. I know of thousands of people who live on such a diet and enjoy extraordinary health. But it also can be modified and changed to adapt to your specific requirements and conditions, your country's customs, your climate, the availability of foods, your health condition, your preferences, etc.

2. Whatever changes you make, keep in mind, however, that the bulk of your diet should consist of seeds, nuts and grains, and fresh vegetables and fruits, preferably organically grown, and up to 80% of them eaten raw. Eat as great a variety of available foods as possible, but not in the same meal, of course. Do not shun potatoes and avocados and bananas because you think they are fattening— they are not!.

3. The menu for lunch and dinner is interchangeable. One big vegetable meal should be eaten at least once a day. If it is eaten for lunch some of the lunch suggestions can be eaten for dinner.

4. Remember, when you eat protein-rich foods (cottage cheese, nuts, beans, etc.) together with carbohydrate-rich foods (salads, fruits, etc.) — eat the protein-rich foods, *first*, or *together with* carbohydrate-rich foods, but not *after*.

5. Do not drink liquids with meals. If thirsty, drink between meals or 15 minutes before meals. Milk or yogurt are foods.

6. If you are taking vitamins and other food supplements, take them *with* meals.

7. One or two tbsp. of brewer's yeast should be taken either with breakfast or lunch, or between meals with fruit juice or yogurt.

8. Finally, follow this Health Menu *every day of your life* and you will live a long life and enjoy the highest possible level of health. And be assured that this Airola Optimum Diet will supply you not only with *all* the vitamins, minerals, essential fatty acids, trace elements, enzymes and the other identified and unidentified nutritive substances, but also with an ade-

quate amount of the highest quality proteins you need for optimum health!

I found Dr. Airola's section of needed supplements in *Are You Confused?* (Published by Health Plus Publishers, P.O. Box 22001, Phoenix, Arizona 85028, $4.95) excellent and am listing them here:

> If you are well, or relatively so, but still wish to supplement your diet for prophylactic reasons, that is, to remain healthy and prevent disease, you should not take concentrated, isolated vitamins, but should use the following foods and food supplements. These supplements will enrich your daily diet and assure you optimum nutrition. They are natural wonder foods, loaded with vital substances. Here they are:
>
> Brewer's Yeast (vitamin B-Complex, protein) 2 or 3 tablespoons each day.Note: never use yeast intended for baking!
>
> Cod Liver Oil, plain, not fortified (vitamins A, F and D) one teaspoon a day.
>
> Raw Wheat Germ (vitamin E, B-complex, protein, minerals, enzymes) 3-5 tablespoons a day. Make sure that ther wheat germ is fresh, not rancid. Fresh wheat germ tastes sweet and does not have a bitter, tangy aftertaste.
>
> Rose Hips, powder or tablets (vitamin C, bioflavonoids, enzymes) equivalent of 200 mg. vitamin C, or more, each day.
>
> Wheat Germ Oil (vitamin E, unsaturated fatty acids) 2 to 3 teaspoons a day.
>
> Bone Meal, powder or tablets (minerals) 2 teaspoons or 10 tablets a day. (Lacto-vegetarians can use Calcium Lactate.)
>
> Kelp (iodine, minerals, trace elements) 2 to 5 tablets a day. Use kelp granules on salads as a substitute for salt.
>
> Lecithin, granules or liquid (inositol, choline, lecithin) 1 tablespoon a day.
>
> For best biological value and most efficient assimilation, all food supplements should be taken with meals. Because some vitamins interfere with the absorption of others, wheat germ oil should be taken before meals and all of the other supplements during or after the meals.

Health Food Stores, Organic Restaurants, A Movement Grows

The current movement toward self-improvement will spur and heighten the expanding number of health food stores sprouting everywhere. Along with this movement is a growing number of excellent natural and organic restaurants which can teach us the joys of wholesome, nutritious eating. Most of these commercial establishments take it upon themselves to *educate* their clientel and are filled with the latest magazines and books on good nutrition. It's difficult to know exactly what and who to believe. You simply have to use discretion and start your own program of self-study and self-analysis. There is no *one way* for everyone. All the faddists and cultists believe they have the answer for everyone else.

It stands to reason that if you are biochemically unique, your nutritional program must be individually developed along with your lifestyle changes. Most health food stores usually offer commodities which are quantum leaps ahead of what you can buy in a regular supermarket and I recommend that you seek them out and begin the journey toward natural health and good food.

Prelude to
Your Spine,
Structural Alignment,
and Flexibility

The next time you are in a crowd, take a close look at the body alignment of those around you. One of the first things you will notice is that almost everyone you see has the head tilted forward. This represents a 10 to 15 pound weight being pulled down by gravity and results in a misalignment of the rest of the body. There is a concave curve in the back that causes the chest and many internal organs to be cramped. This adversely affects both breathing and moving and, more subtly, the person's self-image.

Bill is one of my clients whose life was significantly changed by the application of alignment and flexibility principles.

> When I was young, I heard a lot about good posture: chest out, shoulders back. This was the ideal. It required quite a lot of effort and as I grew older I gave it up. I hardly considered posture for the next 30 years or so. Then one day I was in a bookstore and was attracted to a book called *Bioenergetics* by Alexander Lowen. I leafed through and skimmed some of the material. He was talking about how we develop holding patterns in certain parts of our body. These holding patterns represent areas of tension. He specifically mentioned the shoulders, the abdomen, and the knees.
>
> Over the next few weeks, I started to monitor these parts of my body. Sure enough, I noticed that if I consciously tried to relax my shoulders and abdomen, I would feel a tremendous difference. I realized that I held my shoulders in a tight fashion most of the time and that I exerted a lot of effort holding my abdomen in. I also noticed that I tended to stand with

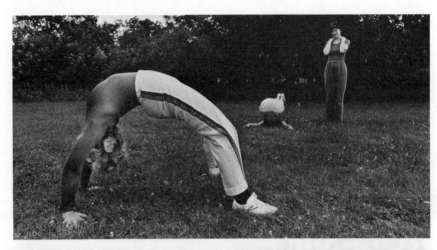

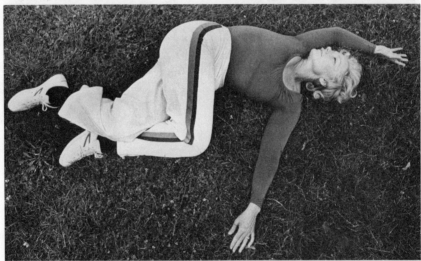

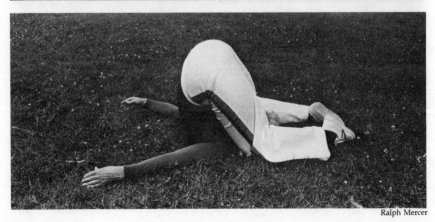

Ralph Mercer

my knees locked. I began to do some of the bioenergetic exercises and these parts of my body loosened up. I would check in on these areas several times each day and consciously relax them. I soon noticed a turnaround. I began to find that most of the time my shoulders were loose, my abdomen relaxed and my knees unlocked.

Then I started to watch what would happen when I would get into a tense situation. My shoulders would tighten and slowly rise. I would unconsciously pull in my abdomen. My knees would shift to a locked position and my breathing would nearly stop. Whenever I would find myself in this situation, I would attempt to relax the areas. I could feel the shoulders drop at least an inch. The abdomen would just drop. I worked on this for almost a year. I was really relaxed but I didn't feel good about my overall posture.

When Dyveke began coaching me, she recommended rolfing. I had read about the process. I had seen "before and after" pictures of people who had been rolfed. There certainly was a difference between the way they stood before the rolfing and afterwards. I had heard a lot about rolfing as it applied to emotional and muscle release. I was basically interested in it from the standpoint of helping my posture. I'll never forget the first session.

I lay on a table while the rolfer, Dr. Gladys Mann, worked on me. She started in the chest area. I relaxed into the burning sensations she created by rubbing her hands across my chest. As she worked on the upper right side of my chest, she said, "Breathe into the area." I did and felt as though my whole chest cavity had been enlarged. The same thing happened on the left side. At the end of the session, I stood up for my *after* picture. My whole chest had opened up. My head also felt very erect.

Gladys said, "Be conscious of how you feel now. Describe it to me." I said, "A little haughty." My chest felt so open and my shoulders were down and relaxed. It wasn't at all like the "shoulders back, chest out" instructions I used to receive as a child. My head was no longer tilted forward. I could feel a lift all along the spinal column. My ears were directly over my shoulders which were over my knees which were over my ankles. It was as if the sections of my body were building blocks and they were perfectly lined up. I felt like aristocracy. "You feel as if you are important. You feel your worth. You don't have to settle for less."

And I realized this was true. I had always had a pretty good self-image, but somehow I felt that, though I knew it, it was not evident to the outside world. Now I felt that my body was telling the whole world that I was more than just another few dollars worth of chemicals. I would not cave in at criticism. I could stand up and take it with the best. In the weeks to come this feedback began to affect me psychologically. It seemed as though I couldn't stand erect and at the same time feel inadequate. My self-image began to change.

This new alignment affected my breathing. Now when I breathe, I breathe more fully. My chest and my abdomen are involved. I no longer have that 15 pounds pulling my whole body forward. Now, my head sits squarely over my body.

As I began to take more notice of my body, I wanted to be able to do things with it. I realized that, even with my good posture, I was somewhat stiff in my movements. I would bend over and be unable to touch the floor. Dyveke recommended a daily workout with some yoga stretching exercises. I found that within a session I could greatly extend my range of motion. I could even begin to put my hands flat on the floor.

The opening up I had felt in the rolfing session had made me want to do some stretches which would open my chest. I found that there are several yoga postures that do this. I remember how proud I felt when I was able to do a bridge, a backward bow, with only my hands and feet on the floor. Soon, I was able to work up to a headstand. Imagine a person 40 years old being able to stand on his head. I had often watched my daughter do it and thought it was just for supple ten-year-olds.

I found that my yoga stretches, when done first thing in the morning, really wake me up and get the cobwebs out of my head. I now begin the day feeling fresh and confident. My body plays an increasingly important part in my life. My flexibility work helps me start the day fully awake, and alive and relaxed and it enables me to do things that I wouldn't have considered before. My alignment reinforces my feeling of self-worth.

I no longer think about slowing down as I get older. I realize that there is no reason I can't move with flexibility, balance, coordination, and pride for the rest of my life.

Chapter Seven:
Your Spine,
Structural Alignment,
and Flexibility

We saw in Chapter Six on nutrition that starting endurance and strength training without first checking out your nutrition was inviting failure in a training program. This chapter represents another of the basics that must precede endurance and strength if you want to minimize discomforts and even serious injuries.

Most car owners know that driving a car with one or more wheels out of balance can do serious damage to the car. For example, it can greatly reduce the life-expectancy of the tires. By the same token, if you begin serious running and strength training on a body that is out of alignment, you are inviting trouble. If you train on a body that has not been preconditioned by stretching the muscles, you invite muscle pulls, tendon tears, etc. And if you conclude a training session without some additional stretching, you are inviting sore, aching muscles.

I can't stress too strongly the importance of to this chapter. The first step is to determine whether you have any serious alignment problems and take care of them before adding endurance and strength training. The second is to always start and end any workout with at least a minimal number of stretches. I also strongly recommend a daily flexibility workout to stretch all parts of your body. Beginning the day with a 20-minute flexibility workout can, as we saw in Bill's case, get your day off of a refreshing start. You might try substituting it for that first cup of coffee.

You will also learn that certain flexibility exercises can bring tension relief during the day. If things get really hectic at the office, take a few minutes to do some stretches and you'll be able to dissipate a lot of tension. If you have to sit for a long time at a desk and you may get back pains. Stop and do some stretches and you'll find you're good for several more hours behind the desk. If you get logy and sleepy during the day, a few flexibility exercises can restore energy to your system.

The Spine

One of the big reasons for flexibility work is to help care for your spine. The spine is nature's switchboard. The messages that go to the organs of your body are transmitted through the spinal cord, through individual spinal nerves, and into a network of trillions of nerve pathways that lead to every cell, every organ, and every tissue of your body.

The spine also is the basic foundation for the bones of your body, your skeletal framework. The spine provides the points of attachment for your ribs, supports your upper arms and your head, allows you to bend and twist, and helps your body absorb shocks that might otherwise jar vital organs.

The importance of the spine is evidenced in its being the very first structure to appear when you are just an embryo in your mother's womb. From that moment on, messages are carried by the trillions as you grow and develop into a full-fledged human being. And once you're born, your spine remains the most important structure in your entire body. Without it and the controlling impulses it channels, nothing would work right. Your stomach wouldn't know what to do with food. Your eyes might develop on your fingertips. Your glands would be out of control.

The 26 bones of the spinal column, called vertebrae, are stacked together to form a protective pathway through which the spinal cord passes. In between the vertebrae, tiny spinal nerves leave the cord at various points to communicate vital nerve energy to various parts of the body. The vertebrae protect the cord from harmful external forces. But this protective covering can also become a hazard. Because the spine must be flexible, each vertebra must be able to move independently. Ideally, after you bend or twist, each veterbra should also be able to return to its proper position.

As long as the spine remains in its normal and natural position, messages are transmitted properly, the body works right, and you enjoy radiant good health. But let just one vertebra move out of line with its neighbors, putting a little bit of pressure on just one tiny nerve, and you experience a reduction of health. This reduction may be unnoticeable to you at the time but certainly can be serious.

Each tiny interference with proper nerve flow can cause a few cells, or an entire organ, to malfunction. If just a few cells are affected, the trouble may not show up immediately. If an entire organ is affected, you may experience discomfort or even pain. In either case, there is a reduction in health. Your *natural* bodily functions will no longer function naturally.

The longer this condition exists, the further you'll go down the road to poor health. And the further you travel this road, the longer it will take your body to recover once the interference is removed.

Your spinal column or vertebral column is a series of movable bones located in the center of your back. There are seven cervical vertebrae (neck), twelve thoracic vertebrae (mid back), and five lumbar vertebrae (low back). These vertebrae are stacked up like building blocks, and between them are located fibrocartilages or disks. These disks help to cushion shock, reduce friction, and allow movement to occur. See Figure One.

So it is important to take care of the spine by doing flexibility work every day, and to have the spine checked from time to time for alignment problems by a professional. Proper care of your spine takes daily awareness and training.

One of the best series of spinal stretches I know of is the ten-step procedure described in Chapter Four in the section on "Creative Running."

I find that the area of alignment and flexibility is a blind spot for many people. This is especially true of the group typified by a male who has gotten into fitness through team sports or individual fitness pursuits such as running. Many of the latest books and magazine articles on running stress the importance of flexibility, especially when warming up and cooling down. But many men have a hard time seeing the relevence of stretching and flexibility. They want to "get on with it." Stretching is just too much trouble for them.

What they fail to realize is that while inaction can lead to muscles rigidity, exercises such as running and weight training can lead to the tightening and shortening of muscles. In weight training, this can result in a condition called *muscle bound*. Running without proper alignment and regular flexibility work can lead to general aching sensations in the body and to serious injuries such as pulled or torn muscles. Thus for people using running as the endurance portion of their Lifestyle Training Program, structural alignment and flexibility are not *options*, they are *necessities*. Failure to take them into account can jeopardize your Lifestyle Training Program and even lead to serious injuries that will deny you the benefits of the program.

Structural Alignment

Imagine a person running several miles a day with his right foot pointed out about 15 degrees. This person will have to make some adjustment to the normal movement of the foot, lower leg, and knee on each footplant. The normal footplant will cause one type of movement, the twisted footplant another. At some point this adjustment will probably lead to leg and knee problems.

Most people try to keep the wheels on their car aligned. But how many ever think of keeping their bodies aligned? It hurts me to see people in

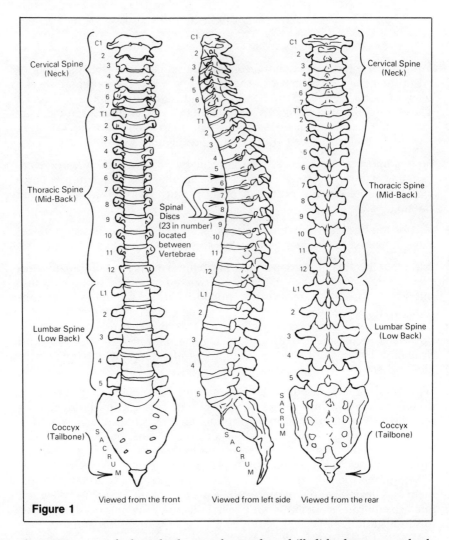

Figure 1

Viewed from the front   Viewed from left side   Viewed from the rear

their 40s start to feel washed up and on a downhill slide due to poor body alignment. And I sometimes want to cry when I see athletes who must have knee or back operations, or who must train in incredible pain because their bodies are out of alignment. I worked with one very knowledgeable medical man who is also a runner. His body was terribly out of alignment. He knew all about tendonitis, heart rate, endurance training, but had never even considered his alignment problem.

In my daily work, I can't believe the number of intelligent, sophisticated, well-educated, professional people who have no concept of the importance of structural alignment in terms of maintaining overall health and preventing disease and injury.

It is crucial to build your training program on a sound base, an aligned body. As far as I'm concerned, *a structurally aligned body is the foundation of physical fitness*. One of the very first steps in a Lifestyle Fitness Program should be to check out the alignment of your body. This ranks with getting the proper shoes in terms of top priority.

Becoming Aware of Your Alignment

You can get some preliminary information about your alignment by observing some things about yourself. It will help to have a friend give you a hand.

First, walk toward a mirror and then just stand naturally and comfortably.

1. Do your feet point pretty much straight ahead or does one or both point in or out?
2. Are both knees pointing straight out? Are your knees locked as far back as they will go? Is one locked and one loose?
3. Are your legs reasonably straight or bowed? Do you tend to stand with one leg further forward than the other?
4. Look at the pelvic area. There should be a little curve in your back, but the pelvis should not be tilted forward or backward.
5. How do your hands hang? Which way are they pointing?
6. Are both shoulders at the same level? Are both in a relaxed position or are they up high with muscles tensed? Are they curved forward or backward?
7. Is your head tilted forward or reasonably erect?
8. What about your spine? Have your friend run his hand up and down your spine from the base of the skull to the bottom of the spine. Are there any vertebrae that protrude outward, inward, or sideways?
9. If you were to look down on your body from above, would the torso be square with your head and legs or would it be twisted? If you ran a plumb line down one side of your body, would your ears be over your shoulders, your shoulders over your hips, your hips over your knees, and your knees over your ankles?

Try jogging at a moderate pace and have your friend observe the plant of your feet. Is there any gross toe-in or toe-out by either foot? Remember one foot may be in alignment while another may be out. Is one shoulder lower than the other? What is the position of your head?

Catch yourself sometimes when you are sitting in a relaxed position. What is your sitting posture like? Are your slumped?

Now check on the aches and pains you sometimes have in your body? Is there a special pain that you get when find yourself in a tense situation e.g., when you realize that you're going to be late for an important appointment? Do you have a chronic pain, say, behind your shoulder blade? Do you have headaches?

Become aware of tensions spots or holding patterns in your body. Are your shoulders tense? Do you forcefully hold your abdomen in?

This inventory can give you clues as to possible alignment problems in your body. It may be that you have certain obvious alignment problems. In this case, you will certainly want to do something about them. And even if there's nothing obvious, you may want to get checked out by a professional. Again, you must take the long view. Your Lifestyle Fitness Program should basically be one you can maintain for the rest of your life. Remember the Biblical example of the house built on a faulty foundation of sand and the house built on a rock. You want your training to be built on the solid foundation of good structural alignment.

Alignment Therapies

There are several body therapies that deal with the problem of structural alignment. Some of these are: yoga, chiropractic, cranial osteopathy, osteopathy, Feldenkrais, and rolfing.

Yoga

I find that people who have had several years of Hatha Yoga, the yoga of physical posture and breathing, are naturals for my training model since their bodies tend to be supple and they are familiar with the concepts of visualization and innerspace. I don't have to stress the importance of alignment and flexibility to people with such background. Every day they practice some of the yoga stretches. Yoga has helped millions of people find a youthfulness, vitality, longevity, gracefulness, and peace of mind that many of their contemporaries do not have. Simple breathing exercises can increase the capacity for taking in oxygen. Limbering and stretching exercises can keep your muscles from becoming tight and help to release tension.

> Yoga is a step-by-step technique for self-discovery and awareness. The initial system of Yoga, which is practiced as a preparation for many of the more meditative and intellectual schools, is called Hatha Yoga. The word *Hatha* consists of two syllables: *Ha* (sun) and *Tha* (moon). In the science of Hatha Yoga, the right side of the body is the positive, male, sun, heat side. The left side is the female, negative, moon, cool side. The word *yoga* means "to join together" or "to yoke."

> Through the practice of Hatha Yoga, the two sides of the body and their characteristic forces are brought into perfect balance. By maintaining this balance, one attains physical health, mental clarity, and steady strength of mind and character.

Yoga asanas or postures are designed to give maximum flexibility and strength to the skeletal, muscular, and nervous systems. The *central nervous system* is composed of the spinal cord and brain. The *peripheral nervous system* is made up of the motor and sensory nerves outside the central nervous system. The autonomic nervous system is made up of the sympathetic and parasympathetic nervous systems and controls the unconscious and involuntary functions of the body and mind.

Yoga exercises lay great stress on the effects of having a very supple, strong back and spinal column. The thousands of nerves which control all organs and areas of the body can be traced to the gigantic network of nerves in the spine and brain. We need to begin at the top of the spine and work through the body by stretching, twisting, balancing, and breathing in a specifically designed manner. Through this process the vital organs are massaged and blood circulation is increased.

This gentle, systematic pressure on the glands and vital organs causes hormones to be secreted. These hormones change the chemistry of the blood. This, in turn, causes a balanced chemical change in the brain which alleviates tension and stress.

Yoga should be practiced in a gentle and systematic way, with great awareness. You should never exceed your limitations. Work up to the more difficult postures. Be regular in your practice of yoga. Set aside 15 to 20 minutes every day. (From *Light of Yoga* by Christensen and Rankin)

The practice of yoga is one way to bring your body into structural alignment. But it will require many years of work to take care of serious structural alignment problems.

Chiropractic

When chiropractic was first introduced to the world in 1895, it involved a new and different approach to the problems of health. The approach up to that time was concerned with specific diseases such as gastritis, headaches, ulcers, colitis, and other disorders. Logically, people tended to ask questions about such specific diseases.

The health care treatment by other doctors consisted primarily of putting chemicals into the body or using drugs in an attempt to restore the body to health. On the other hand, the chiropractic profession and its drugless approach to health maintained that the body receives all the chemicals it needs to achieve good health through the food we eat, the oxygen we breathe, and the water we drink. This new science emphasized that when disease occurred, it was because the body was failing to digest, absorb, circulate, or metabolize food chemicals properly or to properly, eliminate wastes from the body.

Figure Two is taken from the latest edition of Gray's *Anatomy*, a standard textbook recognized by all medical colleges and widely used in the leading schools of medicine, osteopathy, and chiropractic. It shows the nerve supply to the vital organs from the brain and spinal cord and demonstrates the need for maintaining uninterrupted communication through the nerves.

The figure helps to explain that every vital organ in the body is connected with and controlled by nerves from the spinal cord and brain. Through this knowledge one can fully understand why chiropractic treatments can relieve so many human ailments.

Until recent years, chiropractors have not found much acceptance among the more traditional medical practitioners. The general public, until more recently, has been divided into camps: those who experienced relief and cures to longstanding illnesses and injuries the medical profession was unable to help, and those who believed the chiropractors were quacks. This conflict has been fostered by a lack of information about the nature of chiropractic and its significance in terms of lifetime optimal health. Some of the resistance to chiropractic has been professional elitism. With the national awareness moving toward an acceptance of more natural healing techniques without surgery and drugs, and a resurgence of interest in fitness and sports, chiropractic is now the second largest therapy in the world. I consider it one of the most valuable and accessible therapies to facilitate sports training in the New Age.

Chiropractic has been defined as "the art of manually adjusting the segments of the spine to allow the nervous system to function free of nerve interference." It is a science, philosophy, and art of the natural wisdom of the body. Chiropractors believe that improper structure will lead to improper function.

According to Dr. Stephen Brown of Cambridge, Massachusetts, my chiropractor on the East Coast, "Chiropractic treatments help the body to heal by realigning the spine and thus correcting not only structural misalignments but the central nervous system."

> The nervous system controls all of the bodily functions from the brain to the tissue cell, and when there is a clear passageway there will be proper function. If there are imbalances in the spine, these nerve impulses will be interfered with. Most people feel aches and pains in their back due to a pinching of the nerve from a vertebrae out of place. There can also be pinching of the nerves that are not pinching on the nerve pain fibers, but pinching on other fibers, since there are 300,000 nerve cells for each spinal nerve. If one of those or a few of those nerve cells are not pain fibers, they are other fibers that go into your liver or intestines or pancreas and cause those organs not to function properly. It's the job of the chiropractor to remove the interference with the nervous system and correct it, thereby giving structural balance and proper function.

> When the bones of the spine are out of alignment, they can be guided back into their proper positions with the help of a skilled chiropractor. With careful analysis, a chiropractor can tell just when your body needs that gentle push. With the aid of a skillfully delivered force, your body can return the out-of-place vertebra to its proper position. Pressure on the nerve is relieved, the nerve is once more able to transmit its messages, and the organ or cell once more receives proper instructions.

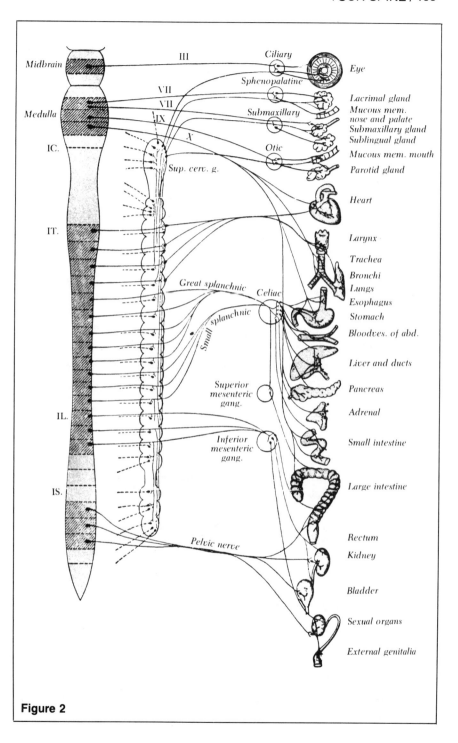

Figure 2

Some of you may not be familiar with the similarities, differences, and overlap between chiropractic and osteopathy (discussed below). Dr. Stephen Brown is trained in a speciality of chiropractic called *cranial osteopathy*. I had a number of these very delicate treatments and asked Dr. Brown to describe the nature of cranial osteopathy.

> Cranial osteopathy was discovered in the 1920's, and recently more chiropractors are becoming specialists in this field and incorporating it into their practice as I do. It was developed by Dr. Sutherland, an osteopathic doctor. He discovered that there was cranial motion. Before that, people believed the skull was solid bone with no motion. This is a key notion, that in order for there to be life there has to be motion. It doesn't matter what part of the body one refers to, the body is not one solid piece in any area. It is fluid. So the cranium, until you die, has motion. When there is no motion, there's death.
>
> There are eight different bones in the skull, 14 different bones in the face, and they are all connected with sutures. There are adjoining points for these different bones and the sutures are beveled in a special way. Everybody has a different interlocking of these bones, just as everyone has different fingerprints.

At this point, Dr. Brown reached backwards and showed me a skull. He held it with the hands of an artist as he pointed out the sutures, connecting bones, and connection to the spinal column. He continued:

> You can see how beautiful and magnificent these sutures are. They're very complex and complicated. They are beveled in a certain way to allow for *motion*. This motion allows for proper brain function.
>
> The brain in not one piece of static material: it pulsates, breathes in and out, and secretes hormones. It's a very fluid organ. The brain expands when you breathe in and contracts when you breathe out. We have to have cranial motion in order to have proper brain function. Cerebral spinal fluid flows from the brain all the way down the spinal cord to the sacrum at the base of the spine. The sacrum pumps while we breathe and forces cerebral spinal fluid back up the spinal cord and into the brain. The cortex of the brain continues to manufacture cerebral spinal fluid.
>
> The cerebral spinal fluid is what bathes the nervous system and the brain in whatever life-giving source it has. In order for the nerves to function properly we have to have continual motion of the cerebral spinal fluid. The motion at the sacrum and the skull must move properly for the proper nerve function. The skull is not one solid lollipop, it's an intricate mechanism with motion. By manipulating this subtle motion in the skull, the body can be realigned and proper nerve function restored.

I asked Dr. Brown about the importance of chiropractics for sports training. He replied:

> A chiropractor deals not only with the nervous system but with muscular imbalances. Athletes are more prone to injuries. Their muscles must have proper tone and strength. When the neuro-muscular junction is firing properly and the nervous system is working as a unit, when the body is structurally balanced, there's less chance of an injury.

The body is held in balance by the antagonist muscles pulling equally against each other. When the muscles are not functioning in an equal manner, stress develops at the joint site, and easy injury is always possible. The constant stress at a joint such as the knee, illustrated in Figure Three (left), causes knee pain; over a long period of time it will cause osteoarthritis, the wear and tear type of arthritis, to develop. If the imbalance is present in a young child, the joint will actually change shape, causing a knock-knee or bow-leg involvement from the abnormal joint shape. An individual who is constantly spraining an ankle is probably the victim of imbalanced muscles in the lower portion of the leg, which hold the ankle in balance.

Many nagging low back pains are a result of the postural balance shift caused by weakening of some muscles and too much contraction of other muscles, illustrated in Figure Three (right). Many so-called "clumsy" children are really victims of muscular imbalance, causing movement to be difficult and uncoordinated.

In my experience as a New Age Coach, some athletes know these principles. Most don't. At the professional, scholastic, and lay public levels, there are a tremendous number of injuries because these principles are not more widely recognized and taught.

In sum, chiropractic is based on the law of homeostasis. That law states that all organisms, when they begin existence, have the ability to maintain themselves and to perform those functions which will ensure their survival, without educated external stimulation, inhibition, etc. The same intelligence which allows a single fertilized egg to grow, differentiate, and develop into a human being is also capable of maintaining that body in a state of health. Disease in not the cause of poor health. Rather, poor health weakens the body so that its structures finally give way and collapse, producing disease.

The law of homeostasis applies to our body's internal functioning. The term we use to discuss this organization is *innate organization or intelligence*. It is this understanding of the universe and the law of homeostasis which breeds the chiropractic philosophy. Chiropractors try to find interference with harmonious function and eliminate it so that the individual can return to normal functioning, a homeostatic state.

Dr. William Baeza, my long-time chiropractor in San Francisco, to whom I am eternally grateful for restoring my health through years of athletic injuries, has often said, "It's so simple, so incredibly simple. Adjust a bone and put it back in place and the life force just flows. People simply get better."

Over the years, many sports-related injuries of my clients have been improved and healed through the use of chiropractics to realign the spinal column. I can't stress enough the importance of seeking regular treatment for care of the spine and daily maintenance through flexibility exercises. Chiropractic is certainly an area that can't be ignored.

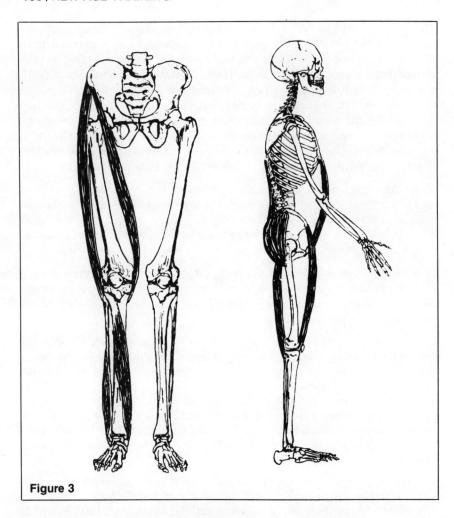

Figure 3

Strengthening Exercises

The two weakest areas of the body, the two most prone to injury, are the lower back and neck. It is important to give special care to these areas through strengthening exercises.

Basic Low Back Exercises

Figure Four shows six low back exercises. The exercises should be done on a firm padded surface such as a carpeted floor. If it is difficult getting down and up from the floor initially, a firm bed might be preferred. A small pillow under the head is sometimes more comfortable.

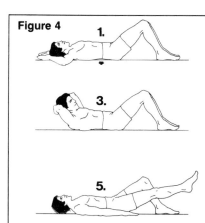

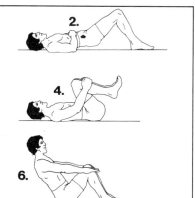

Figure 4

1. The basic starting position for all the exercises is lying on your back with the knees bent and the back flat against the floor. Tighten the muscles of the abdomen and buttocks at the same time to force and firmly flatten your back against the floor. Hold for 5 to 10 seconds. Relax and repeat 5 to 10 times.

2. Assume the basic starting position. Raise the hips off the floor about 6 inches and tighten the muscles of the hips and buttocks. Hold for 5 to 10 seconds. Relax back down on the floor and repeat 5 to 10 times.

3. Assume the basic starting position with hands behind the head. Raise your head off the floor while forcefully contracting the abdominal muscles. A loud grunt of "AAAHH" is helpful in doing this exercise to prevent internal pressure. Relax to starting position and repeat 5 to 10 times.

4. Assume the basic starting position. Bring both knees to the chest, grabbing your knees with your hands and pulling your knees toward your chest as close as possible. Hold for the count of 10. Relax back to the starting position and repeat 5 to 10 times.

5. Assume the basic starting position. Extend one leg straight out. Raise the straight leg about 6 inches off the floor and hold for 5 to 10 seconds. Return to the starting position with both knees bent. Repeat the movement with the opposite leg. Repeat the exercise 5 to 10 times.

6. This exercise should not be done until the other exercises have been done for several weeks. Assume the basic starting position. Pull up to a sitting position, being certain to keep the knees bent. It is helpful to put the feet under a heavy chair or sofa for support, or have someone hold the feet to the floor.

Start the exercises slowly and gently. Never overdo exercising. Allow the muscles to loosen up. Mild heat or a hot tub soak for five to ten minutes just before starting can help relax tight muscles.

1. The basic starting position for all the exercises is lying on your back with the knees bent and the back flat against the floor. Tighten the muscles of the abdomen and buttocks at the same time to force and firmly flatten your back against the floor. Hold for 5 to 10 seconds. Relax and repeat 5 to 10 times.

2. Assume the basic starting position. Raise the hips off the floor about 6 inches and tighten the muscles of the hips and buttocks. Hold for 5 to 10 seconds. Relax back down on the floor and repeat 5 to 10 times.

3. Assume the basic starting position with hands behind the head. Raise your head off the floor while forcefully contracting the abdominal muscles. A loud grunt of "AAAHHH" is helpful in doing this exercise to prevent internal pressure. Relax to starting position and repeat 5 to 10 times.

4. Assume the basic starting position. Bring both knees to the chest,

grabbing your knees with your hands and pulling your knees toward your chest as close as possible. Hold for the count of 10. Relax back to the starting position and repeat 5 to 10 times.

5. Assume the basic starting position. Extend one leg straight out. Raise the straight leg about 6 inches off the floor and hold for 5 to 10 seconds. Return to the starting position with both knees bent. Repeat the movement with the opposite leg. Repeat the exercise 5 to 10 times.

Exercises for the Neck

Figure Five shows a series of six exercises for the neck. Do each of the exercises three to five times, preferably twice a day. The exercises should be done slowly and gently. Do not force the motions of the head and neck beyond the point of pain.

1. Hunch your shoulders up high and rotate in a circular motion forward, then reverse and rotate the shoulders backwards.

2. Gently bend the head forward, attempting to touch the chin to the chest.

3. Gently bend the head backwards to its limit.

4. Bend the head to the right as far as possible.

5. Bend the head to the left as far as possible.

6. Carefully roll the head around in a wide circle in one direction, then reverse and roll the head around in the opposite direction.

Remember that the key to joint dysfunction is flexibility and mobility. It is impossible to obtain normal range of motion of the neck without proper exercise.

The neck region described earlier demonstrates some of the weaknesses of the spine. A typical example of a common injury to the neck region is illustrated in the rear-end auto collision. (See Figure Six.) The driver, not expecting such an incident, is relaxed. The force from behind causes the head to flip quickly backwards and then thrust forward by the deceleration (quick stopping) motion.

This type of rapid movement and the manner in which the head is thrust about has been termed *whiplash*. Many injuries of this nature are not immediately felt by the injured person. Authorities estimate that the injuries may not be felt for several hours to years following the incident.

Whiplash is the common name given to an injury in which there is a hyper-flexion (increased forward motion), hyper-extension (increased backward motion) injury to the cervical (neck) spine. The reason for that particular name is due to the fact that the spine is held in place in the mid-back by the attachment of the rib cage. In any movement, therefore, to which the spine may be subjected, as in the case of an auto accident, or severe fall, the neck is the area most commonly injured.

EXERCISES FOR THE NECK

Do each of the exercises three to five times, preferably twice a day. The exercises should be done slowly and gently. Do not force the motions of the head and neck beyond the point of pain.

Remember that the key to joint dysfunction is flexibility and mobility. It is impossible to obtain normal range of motion of the neck without proper exercise.

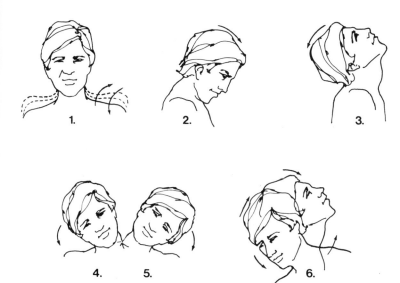

1. Hunch your shoulders up high and rotate in a circular motion forward, then reverse and rotate the shoulders backwards.

2. Gently bend the head forward attempting to touch the chin to the chest.

3. Gently bend the head backwards to its limit.

4. Bend the head to the right as far as possible.

5. Bend the head to the left as far as possible.

6. Carefully roll the head around in a wide circle in one direction, then reverse and roll the head around in the opposite direction.

Figure 5

Some examples of this type of reaction from an injury of this nature could be: Headaches, visual disturbance, stiffness of the neck, restriction of movement, shoulder, neck and arm pain, neuralgia, etc.

Prompt attention to this type of trauma can help to avoid many of the symptoms which could develop at a later date.

(The discussion in this section is based in part on Dr. Louis Sportelli's booklet *Introduction to Chiropractic*, the finest reference work I have seen on this subject.)

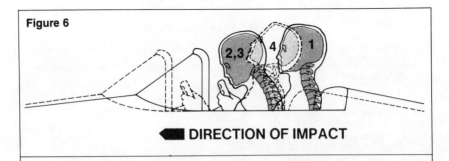

Figure 6

DIRECTION OF IMPACT

WHIPLASH INJURY (Hyper Extension • Hyper Flexion)

1. IMPACT FROM THE REAR
2. BODY THROWN FORWARD (Head remains stationary, appearing to move backward)
3. SIDE NECK MUSCLES TIGHTEN (Sternocleidomastoids) SNAPPING HEAD FORWARD (Tearing muscles)
4. HEAD RETURNS TO NORMAL POSITION (Leaving cervical spine and muscle damage)
5. THE RESULT — DISTORTION OF THE NATURAL CERVICAL CURVE

Osteopathy

Osteopathy is a school of medicine that deals with the whole person. An osteopathic doctor attends a medical school and uses all the modalities of medicine including drugs and surgery, but also uses manipulative therapies. Such a doctor first tries to help the body treat itself rather than give medicines or use other forms of treatment. Osteopaths treat all areas of the body in all positions when performing their manipulative treatments on the skeletal muscle frame.

There are about 18,000 osteopathic doctors in the United States, and 15 medical schools to train such practitioners. Osteopathy is growing very rapidly. According to Dr. Charles Lowney, of Arlington, Massachusetts, 75 percent of the graduates of traditional medical schools go into some medical specialty. It is just the opposite with osteopathic doctors. Seventy-five percent become general practitioners, for they believe the real need is in family practice, treating the whole person and the whole body from a preventive point of view.

I asked Dr. Lowney about the importance of osteopathy with the surging interest in sports, running and fitness. He said:

> I see a lot of runners with low back and foot problems. They believe the problem is in the back and foot. The problem is, however, a *structural one*. The body's frame is out of alignment, affecting the pressure and balance of the hips, knees, legs, and ankles. Good structural alignment prevents and avoids injuries. Healthy structure promotes normal functioning. Abnormal functioning causes back problems, especially lower

back problems. The more healthy the structure of the body, the more healthy the person's entire system."

Every state has an Association for Osteopathic Physicians which can be located in a telephone book. The number of these doctors is growing and, as they assume an increasingly prominent place in society, the general public will come to understand that optimal health is basically a matter of self-knowledge and self-regulation. Optimal health must be built upon a structurally aligned and balanced skeletal muscle frame.

Feldenkrais

Feldenkrais exercises were developed by Israeli-born Dr. Moshe Feldenkrais. Not only is Dr. Feldenkrais a physicist but a mathematician and former champion black-belt in judo. Following a knee injury and the recommendation of surgery, Dr. Feldenkrais rejected surgery and instead developed a system of exercises that re-train the awareness of the body with respect to movement. His book *Awareness Through Movement* contains an outstanding synthesis of his life's work and closes with specific exercises to increase one's range of motion. Not only do these exercises teach *awareness*, they can also have a profound effect on altering one's self-image. As he states:

> The ability to move is important to self-value. A person's physical build and his ability to move are probably more important to his self-image than anything else.

> Movements reflect the state of the nervous system and movement is the basis of awareness. Most of what goes on within us remains dulled and hidden from us until it reaches the muscles. We know what is happening within us as soon as the muscles of our face, heart, or breathing apparatus organize themselves into patterns known as fear, anxiety, laughter, or any other feeling.

The Feldenkrais exercises are slow-moving and meditative, designed to break fixed patterns of movement and allow the skeletal muscles a greater range of flexibility. The significance of this pioneering work in lifestyle fitness and sports training is enormous. As Feldenkrais states:

> The reason why we should choose the action-system at the point of attack for the improvement of man is because all behavior is a complex of mobilized muscles, sensing, feeling and thought. The part played by the muscles is so large that if it were omitted from the patterns in the motor cortex the rest of the components of the pattern would disintegrate.

> The motor cortex of the brain, where patterns activating the muscles are established, lies only a few millimeters above the brain strata dealing with association processes. All the feeling and sensing that a man has experienced were at one time linked with the association processes.

> Muscles play the main role in awareness. Owing to the close proximity to the motor cortex of the brain structures dealing with thought and feeling, and the tendency of processes in brain tissue to diffuse and spread to

neighboring tissues, a drastic change in the motor cortex will have parallel effects on thinking and feeling. (*Awareness Through Movement*, Moshe Feldenkrais, pp. 34-36)

Thus, changing one's ability to increase the range of motion with new awareness can not only exert profound emotional changes, but can alter one's self-concept. This accounts for the emotional releases and increased sensitivity that often emerges when one is performing a Feldenkrais exercise. Sports training in the New Age is meant to awaken us to feelings and inner awareness, to heighten our sensitivity to subtleties and expand our sense of self. There is no system of exercises more conducive to fulfilling these requirements than Feldenkrais.

Dr. Feldenkrais has also developed a system of body therapy whereby a trained practitioner moves another person's body to *teach* through motor-learning how to extend movement patterns or correct faulty, limiting ones. This procedure shortens the time it takes to facilitate an increased range of motion when compared with taking classes and doing the exercises under direction. Practitioners of this system of body manipulation undergo intensive training with Dr. Feldenkrais, and at the present there are only a very few in the world.

Dr. Feldenkrais conducts regular training sessions to develop teachers. He also conducts classes for up to two hundred at a time in large halls. He is a dramatic, charismatic person, sometimes volatile and impatient. As a student, one learns to accept his unique personality, and he is always surrounded by an entourage of adoring devotees. At the present time, classes in this technique are more difficult to find than classes in yoga. A local growth center or holistic health center usually knows their location.

At the Esalen Sports Center, we were instrumental in introducing the amazing effects of these exercises both to seasoned athletes and the lay public in a series of national conferences. I have had many personal experiences with Dr. Feldenkrais both as student and client. He has worked on my body to teach me new and improved neurological functioning. Several of his assistants, notably Ruth Alon, have corrected imbalances with gentle corrective manipulations.

There is a special quality about his work that has a devotional, perhaps spiritual quality. One feels deep respect for the natural wisdom and feedback of the body sense. There is no attempt to interfere, only to guide lovingly to a different, expanded awareness.

The nature and quality of Feldenkrais exercises are not such that they can be condensed in this book. Dr. Feldenkrais has high standards of excellence and certification and rightly wants his work carried by responsible and legitimate teachers. His book gives 12 beginning lessons that anyone can do. Cassette tapes of specific exercises can be ordered from Esalen Institute, Big Sur, California. Perhaps describing an experience will give you a better idea of the nature of this work.

At the Esalen Sports Center Summer Training Institute, Betty Fuller, a certified instructor, was leading us through a three-day session. I was lying on my back with one knee crossed over the other. My arms were extended straight out, away from my body, and my fists were closed. Betty was cajoling us with a soft voice. I was in some dreamlike state of relaxation but with great awareness. Slowly, over a 45-minute period of time, I was guided to rotate my fist forward, then backwards, let my crossed legs gently fall to the right or left side and my head do likewise. I was instructed to move my eyes in the opposite direction to the position of my head.

The fifth rotation in the series opened up the range of motion in my shoulder sockets and the crossed-knee rotaton opened up the range of motion in the pelvic area. All during the session, although "awake", I was so relaxed that my consciousness was only focused on the delight of the delicacy and subtlety of sensing the increased mobility I was feeling.

As I stood up, after 45 minutes, a radiant feeling of peace, balance and harmony thrilled me. There was a bursting feeling inside. I knew some remarkable release had taken place.

I have seen the same results so many times in my years of traveling and teaching that it no longer surprises me. I consider Dr. Feldenkrais a great inventor and pioneer. He has devoted his lifetime to developing this remarkable tool of natural healing. In these exercises, he prepares us to live in a pain-free, mobile, flexible body that moves with awareness.

Rolfing

Probably the quickest and most effective treatment for alignment problems is *rolfing*, also known as structural alignment. One of the main purposes of rolfing is to bring the various parts of the body, the head, shoulders, thorax, pelvis and legs, into a vertical axis. This allows gravity to exert a positive influence on the body rather than the negative one that results when one or more of these body segments is out of alignment. When the body segments are in alignment, the skeleton and muscles can properly support weight. In a misaligned state, there is a strained imbalance with an attendant tension that results in the shortening of the muscles and tissues that connect them. Rolfing helps to bring these tissues back to their normal state, which in turn frees the body segments for proper alignment and movement.

The nature of the work requires a practitioner to exert pressure on the body while following the line of connective tissue. Imagine a thumb or knuckle pressed from your wrist up to your elbow. Some people experience pain during rolfing. It is important to relax the mind and allow the new *body sense* to take over. I personally did not experience pain except for very brief moments, and even then felt corrective and therapeutic.

Rolfing is meant to produce more efficient use of muscles and also decrease the energy required to use them. It is accomplished by a series of ten one-hour sessions.

Ida Rolf describes rolfing in a Big Sur Recording.

> When looking at a body, it is a body in an environment, a material aggregate that is operating in an energy field; the field of gravity. The premise of our work in healing, reorganizing bodies and increasing vitality of bodies, depends on the idea that *bodies are unbelievably plastic*. This means that they can be deformed to a great extent, without breaking. Thus, a body can be *reformed* without breaking. It can be reformed because it is a consolidation of segments that stack on top of one another and the whole thing is bound in an elastic sack: a shopping bag.

> These bony segments are held in place by soft muscles and skin. On the basis of this idea, we can change the structure of human beings because that soft elastic tissue can be changed by the addition of energy to it and bones shifted slightly. This is what rolfing is all about. By virtue of this elasticity and the plasticity of soft tissue, we can get bones from where they *don't* belong to where they do *belong*.

> *The body is a series of blocks and must be stabilized and aligned with gravity. This can be facilitated by ten sessions of rolfing to realign the soft tissue and allow the blocks of the body to be properly realigned.*

The following is a description of the third of ten rolfing sessions I experienced with Dr. Ed Jackson of Berkeley, California:

> I lay on my side and Ed's elbow, knuckles, and fingers went into my floating rib to readjust it and correct my upper torso. Each time he probed an area of blocked energy I would relinquish and allow the cells to open to the biting search of healing power. The deep breathing by both Ed and me, a rhythmic harmonic interchange, was interspersed with harmoniously laced pain.

> At times my need for total relinquishment was so intense I almost fell asleep. The sheer exhaustion of trying to make sense of the nonsense of my life pulled my head into the pillow, into the massage table. At one point Ed worked around the fifth lumbar and floods of impressions about hundreds of hours on the tennis court came alive. I could see the way I stopped abruptly for a net shot or backhand and pulled and torqued my body around that spot where the fascia had clumped.

> I mentioned I had been running eight to ten miles up and down Mount Tamalpais and my hamstrings seemed tight. He had me roll over on my back and pull my knees to my chest while his elbows worked down the hamstring and the buttocks. I could feel the connections just below the knees to where a long-time sore spot hid crippling pain. Ed took a moment to show that connection on a wall chart.

> Back on the table, I turned to the other side and was surprised that the left side was tighter than the right. He seemed particularly pleased that he could go in so deep and get the floating rib and readjust it. I felt a slow tilt taking place in my pelvic area. The two previous sessions had brought a total realignment of my hips and legs. No longer did I feel the twinge of pain around the knee sockets each time I ran, or the pull of the

ankle that had been sprained so many times. The whole shifting of the weight of my body had altered my state into one of balance and fluidity. I felt the tuck of the spine and the opening up around the lower lumbar region and the hips, around the vagina and the hamstrings.

A beautiful fountain of energy and warmth started to bubble and erupt, and a shower of vibrant streamers coursed through the sinews and unseen arches holding this intricate machine, my body, together.

Which Therapy Is Best?

Choosing the correct therapy and therapist for you will call for some effort. You will have to do some investigation for yourself. The therapies I have mentioned will give a starting point for your investigation. Often a practitioner of one of the therapies believes that therapy contains the total answer. But I disagree. From my experience, I have found that the various therapies complement and augment each other.

The method that yields the fastest results in term of bringing the various parts of your body into alignment is rolfing. But there are two potential disadvantages. First, rolfing is expensive. It generally involves ten sessions at $40 to $60 each. The ten sessions cover the whole body. I have seen many instances of dramatic changes in body alignment as a result of rolfing. Second, rolfing usually often involves an emotional component. The deep massage work oftens unblocks emotions bound up in the area being rolfed and can bring up deep feelings. Part of the rolfer's training is to help a client deal with these surfacing emotions.

Alignment, especially as it concerns the spine, must be maintained. I personally use chiropractic for this maintainence. Some people wonder why it is necessary to have more than one spinal adjustment. It is necessary because it took years for the misalignment to reach its current stage, and the vertebrae must be slowly worked in place. As this is done, the rest of the spinal column must be adjusted to absorb the realignment.

Yoga and Feldenkrais can both be used to bring the body into better structural alignment but both take longer than rolfing or chiropractic. However, all of the techniques can help keep your alignment stable once some initial corrective work has been done by a trained practitioner.

The technique or techniques you finally choose for correcting any structural problems in your body and maintaining good alignment may depend on what is available in your community, and the interaction you are able to establish with a particular practitioner. I can't emphasize too strongly the value of having a trusted practioner to help you with your alignment problems. As I have said, I can recommend any of the therapies I have discussed. One factor that would lead me to choose a particular one over the others is the level of trust I felt with the practitioner.

As Oyle states in *The Healing Mind*:

> Whatever you put your trust in can be a precipitating agent for your cure. Inner belief is the vital factor in any healing practice regardless of the ritual employed.
>
> Two factors are essential to the therapeutic relationship:
>
> The physician must have complete confidence in his healing system or ritual and the patient must trust that the physician knows what he is doing. If either aspect of this inner belief is missing, the healing process is adversely affected. The healing factor is under the complete control of the psyche which can cause disease or initiate healing.

Strength Training

In my training model, strength is one of the basic components. In order to condition your body so that you may participate more fully in life, you need to include strength training in your Lifestyle Training Program. By systematically strengthening the major muscle sets in your body, you will be able to move faster, farther, and more efficiently when you take long walks, climb mountains, ski, play tennis. You will also protect yourself from injury when you participate in activities involving moving. As Ellington Darden points out in *Strength Training Principles*, strong muscles provide increased joint stability.

The psychological benefits of strength training should not be overlooked either. A person whose body is soft, flabby, and out of shape can't help but be affected by the resulting self-image. Strength training, as part of an overall Lifestyle Training Program, can help the person build a positive self-image that comes from having a firm, sleek body and the knowledge that the body is fully prepared for some of the strenuous activities of life that can make life more fun.

It is my belief that strength training should always be done on an aligned body. So once you have taken care of your body alignment, you will be ready to start your strength training. Darden's small book gives one of the best summaries I've seen on the proper approach to strength training. I have summarized his six principles:

1. Try to increase the workload, the resistance, in every workout. In general, 8 to 12 repetitions per set gives the best results, but with any set keep up the repetitions until further movement is impossible. If you can do more than 8 to 12 repetitions in a set, increase the resistance for that set in the next workout.
2. Strength building depends on the intensity of exercise. The workload must produce a high intensity contraction. Hard work alone seldom produces a significant increase in strength.
3. How you perform the exercise is crucial. Repetitions should be in a slow, smooth manner throughout the entire movement, avoiding

jerking. The range of movement should be as great as possible from full extension to full flexion and should start in a pre-stretching position. The lowering portion of the exercise is more important than the raising.

4. Use exercises that involve the greatest range of movement of the major muscle groups. In each exercise, there should be resistance throughout the whole range of movement: extended, mid-range, and contracted.

5. Your workout should begin with exercises that involve the largest muscle groups and then proceed down to the smaller groups. In each workout, include some form of exercise for each of the major muscle masses of your body.

6. Practice high intensity but brief and infrequent training: one set of each exercise per workout, 30 minutes per session, with a minimum of 48 hours and a maximum of 96 hours between sessions. As you advance in training, you do not need more training but harder training, i.e., higher intensity training.

Most of us think of dumbbells and barbells when we think of strength training. But current research indicates that this form of strength training is not the best way to build strength. One of the major problems is that it is not possible to maintain resistance over the full range of movement. Leverage and strength vary over the range of movement of an exercise and dumbbells and barbells cannot compensate for this variation.

There is a system of weight training available in most areas that is based on the six principles above. It is called Nautilus. The Nautilus equipment is being used by many professional athletes in all sports and is now available to everyone, men and women, who want to increase strength in a safe, efficient, and effective manner.

A Nautilus facility includes a set of machines designed to provide a workout for specific muscle sets, e.g. hip and back, leg extension, leg press, leg curl, pullover, shoulder, neck, chest, and biceps and triceps. When you join Nautilus, a trained instructor guides you through your first few workouts, showing you the proper weight and number of repetitions for each machine. You have a progress card on which you note this information for each machine every time you work out. The emphasis is on having the proper weight so that you can go through the full range of movement for the recommended number of repetitions but no more. The Nautilus machines are geared in such a way that you get variable resistance over the range of movement. You have more leverage at some points in the movement than others, so more resistance is needed at those points. Each machine also provides pre-stretching.

Many Nautilus facilities offer three-month memberships for approximately $90. You can set up your three-workout-per-week schedule to fit your time requirements. If you use the Nautilus machines as they are meant to be used, you will no doubt make more and faster progress than you could with any other available approach.

However, I realize that not everyone will be able to take advantage of Nautilus. Don't let this keep you from including a strength training component in your Lifestyle Training Program because neither endurance training nor flexibility workouts will substitute for strength training.

Whatever you do, become familiar with the principles in Darden's book and then try to set up a strength training procedure that will give you an intense 30-minute workout three days a week. If you have to use conventional weights, try to come as close as possible to applying the six principles above.

One alternative to conventional weights is a device called the *Stretch-Ur*, developed by my friend and student Wayne Lee. The *Stretch-Ur* offers a convenient way to approximate many of the Nautilus benefits with a simple, portable device. Wayne would be the first to tell you that a workout with the Stretch-Ur is not equivalent to a workout at Nautilus, but it may well be superior to conventional weights with much less hassle.

The *Stretch-Ur* is a six-foot length of latex with a handle on each end. A webbed strap is provided to enable you to use a door jamb or heavy piece of furniture to secure the *Stretch-Ur* for many of the exercises.

The *Stretch-Ur* has unusual strength and elasticity. It can be stretched several times its length without breaking or losing its shape. You can increase resistance for a particular exercise simply by moving out farther from the anchor point. This means that you can move quickly from exercise to exercise since you don't have to change weights. The portability of the *Stretch-Ur* makes it especially attractive to a person who travels a lot since it can be folded into a package no larger than two large fists.

Flexibility

Flexibility work is one of the most crucial parts of a Lifestyle Training Program. (I introduced the concept in Chapter 4 in the section "Before the Run: STRRRRETCH!") The spine is the lifeline of the body; through it all body movement flows. Care of the spine is largely neglected in sports. For instance, in tennis, an impact sport, the twisting, bending, jerking and smashing send shockwaves through the body, causing pinched nerves and attendant injuries to internal organs. Often people have to give up the sport. Pulled tendons and tennis elbow are well-known tennis ailments. But all this need not be part of the game.

It is not enough to get your body into alignment. You must work to keep it there. A Lifestyle Training Progam should include some therapies where practitioners work on your body, but ultimately you must be your own guide and discipline your will through affirmations and inspiration to keep an alignment and flexibility ritual established. Maintenance of alignment and flexibility must be seen as essential to the self-management of health.

Testing Your Flexibility

In the first part of the chapter, you did a self-assessment of your alignment. In this section, I will show you how to do a self-assessment of your flexibility. It's fun to take these kinds of tests. But what you must remember is that even if the test shows that you are very flexible right now, you will still need a daily program of exercises to maintain your flexibility, especially if you are about to begin a running program and/or weight training. Flexibility is not a state you attain and then have forever. You must constantly work at it.

Following is a test of flexibility taken from Kounouvsky's research. As you take this test, remember that many things can affect a person's degree of flexibility, among them physical characteristics, state of tension or relaxation and even the surrounding temperature.

1. Shoulders (See Figure Seven)

The smaller the distance between your wrists and the wall, the more supple your shoulders are. If the distance is more than ten inches, your shoulders are pretty stiff and you must avoid exercises involving suspension from a bar or other apparatus until you have improved your flexibility. If you can touch the wall, your shoulder flexibility is good. If you are less than six inches away, it is fair, and over six inches is insufficient.

2. Forward Suppleness of Spine (See Figure Eight)

Sit on the floor, legs together and straight, toes pointed. Bend forward, without forcing, and try to touch your toes with your fingertips.

The distance between your fingertips and toes reflects your forward suppleness. Measure the distance for future reference.

Fingertips overlapping toes is good. Less than ten inches is fair and over ten inches is insufficient.

3. Backward Suppleness of Spine (women) (See Figure Nine)

Note: A man's muscular development usually interferes with the backward flexibility of his spine, but most women, if they are fit, should be able to do this test. It there is a free arch with no pull your backward suppleness is good. If you can get your shoulders and knees ten to 12 inches off the floor, your backward suppleness is adequate. Five inches off the floor is fair. If you have difficulty grasping your ankles, it is insufficient.

4. Lateral Flexibility (See Figure Ten)

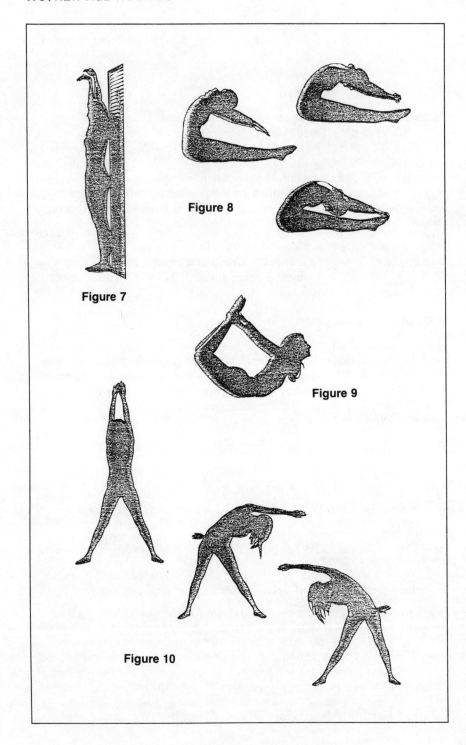

Figure 7

Figure 8

Figure 9

Figure 10

Figure 11

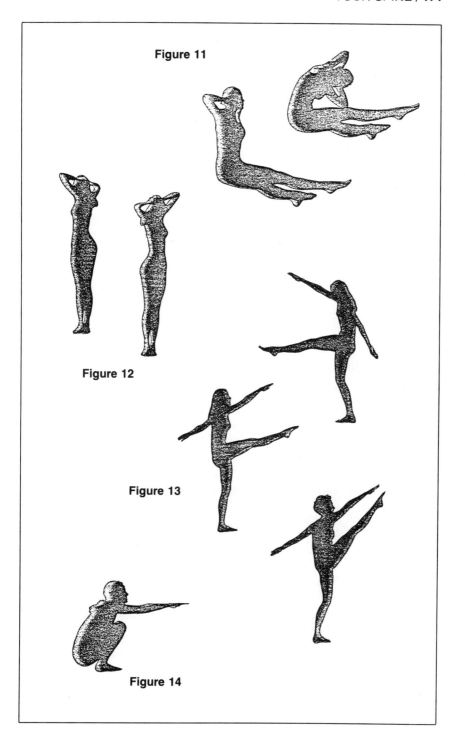

Figure 12

Figure 13

Figure 14

Perform the exercise as if you were sliding against an imaginary wall.

A bend of over 80 degrees is good, 45 to 80 degrees is fair, and less than 45 degrees is insufficient,

5. Twisting (See Figure Eleven)

If you can touch each knee with the appropriate elbow, you are flexible enough. If you cannot, note the distance between knee and elbow. Up to six inches is fair and over six inches is insufficient.

6. Pivoting (See Figure Twelve)

If you can see 180 degrees from each side, i.e., six o'clock, your pivoting suppleness is good. If you can see 120 degrees, i.e., four o'clock when you twist to the right and eight o'clock when you twist to the left, it is fair. Less than 120 degrees is insufficient.

7. Hips (Primarily for Women) (See Figure Thirteen)

Stand and raise your right arm forward, the hand slightly above the level of your head, the other arm back for balance. Swing your right leg forward and try to touch your right hand without bending your knees or lowering your hand. Then try the test with your left arm and leg.

Note the distance between your toes (pointed) and your hands.

8. Hips, Knees, and Ankles (See Figure Fourteen)

If you have complete flexion and an easy position, the suppleness of your hips, knees, and ankles is good. A complete bend holding on to a chair is fair. Inability to reach position is insufficient.

If you cannot perform the above tests with ease and freedom, your suppleness is inadequate. If some of your joints are not supple enough, you will not be able to do certain exercises fully or freely and they will be less effective.

Suppleness has no age limit and only inactivity induces a stiffening of joints and limitation of movement.

Quick and Light Yoga Routines

The following flexibility exercises are taken from *Light of Yoga* by Alice Christensen and David Rankin.

The Quick Routine of Essential Postures   Figure Fifteen (top) shows a set of seven postures for those who have a very busy and demanding schedule but would like a routine that could give good benefits ten to 15 minutes.

The Light Routine   Figure Fifteen (bottom) shows a routine designed for those who have 20 to 25 minutes to spend on an easy work-out. This will provide the essential stretches, twists and balances necessary for good health and clarity of mind, relieving stress for those individuals who have a very demanding schedule. Note that the *Light Routine* includes some of the *Quick Postures* illustrated at the top of Figure Fifteen.

I recommend using at least the *Quick* routine before and after the endurance portion of your training program, e.g., before and after running. They should also be used before and after your strength training.

Four Stretches for the Legs

Runners who do not stretch should not be surprised that their legs feel tight and inflexible when they start to run. They are increasing the chances of tearing a tendon and developing tendonitis. Runners who do not stretch should not be surprised to find that they sometimes wake up in the middle of the night with sore, aching legs. This is the result of insufficient cooldown after a run. If you suddenly stop after running, blood pools in your legs and lactic acid is not cleared. Stretching after a run can help combat this effect.

There is a series of four flexibility exercises recommended by Dr. David Bachman, each of which stretches one of four major muscle sets in the legs: the calf, the hamstring, the adductor, and the quadricep. Dr. Bachman recommends that each stretch be held for five seconds and repeated five times.

These exercises are especially good for beginners in the area of stretching. They are good for developing awareness of the four major muscle sets. When done properly, each stretch produces a slight burning sensation in the affected area. Don't try to exaggerate the burn when stretching, but be able to feel it for the full five seconds.

Don't confuse doing these four stretches with a full flexibility program. There is no stretching of the spinal column here, for example. You will want to move as soon as possible to the quick and then the light yoga stretches shown above while maintaining the stretches in this section.

Stretches for Two or More People

The following are a series of *dead weight* stretches which I evolved and which have sometimes had a profound impact in releasing emotional blocks:

Back on back   Stand back to back with a partner. Bend forward and take the partner onto your back. Encourage the partner to totally let go and relax into you. This exercise stretches the complete spine in reversed position.

Leg Stretch for Two People   Partner 1 faces a tree and bends over with hands near the bottom of the tree. Partner 2 lifts Partner 1's left leg and puts it on

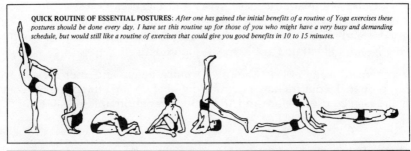

QUICK ROUTINE OF ESSENTIAL POSTURES: *After one has gained the initial benefits of a routine of Yoga exercises these postures should be done every day. I have set this routine up for those of you who might have a very busy and demanding schedule, but would still like a routine of exercises that could give you good benefits in 10 to 15 minutes.*

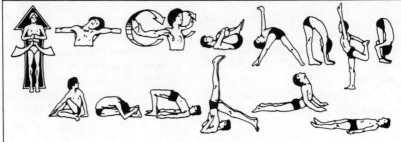

THE LIGHT ROUTINE: *This routine is for those of you who would like to have about 20 to 25 minutes of an easy work-out. This will provide the essential stretches, twists, and balances necessary for good health and clarity of mind, relieving stress for those individuals who have a very demanding schedule but would like to keep up their Yoga practice.*

Figure 15

his or her shoulder. Partner 2 holds the leg gently and instructs partner to relax the leg being held and push back to straighten the opposite leg. The partner whose hands are on the tree, keeps bending lower and lower with tremendous *inner awareness*. Then the same is then done with the opposite legs. Afterwards, allow the partner to walk and feel the spring in his or her legs. Then the partners should exchange positions and repeat the exercise.

I once ran 23 miles from Esalen Big Sur to Nepenthe with Ian Jackson, who first taught me this stretch. It enabled me to run the distance without pain and I have subsequently taught it in all my workshops. I believe it not only releases ligament and tendon binding, but allows the lactic acid buildup to be siphoned off. Besides, it is nurturing and supportive.

Four on One In this exercise, four people lift a fifth off the ground and sway him from side to side. Lift up, drop down, gently undulate the body, pull alternate sides, swing. I have been impressed with the impact that simple techniques of innerspace training and physical exercises can have on personality reorganization. There are breakthroughs of creativity, release of emotional tension and blocks, and moments of inner awareness. This is not surprising considering the connection between the motor cortex of the brain and thinking and feeling, as Dr. Feldenkrais pointed out. The experience of Donna in a workshop is a good example of how these techniques can work.

After some modified spinal stretches, I wanted the group to run. I suggested that they gently open their eyes and then continue to close and open them as they stood up so as to retain this sense of inner peace as they started to connect to their outer reality. The entire group stood up with the exception of Donna, who lay on her side cuddled up. She wasn't crying overtly but I sensed some emotional changes going on inside of her.

I bent down and started to stroke her body lightly, and within moments signaled three men to come and help me pick her up. We each took a leg or arm, and Donna seemed to feel that she was going to experience something new, and she seemed to just go with the flow. Gently we lifted her body and started to sway her from side to side, in rhythm with a set of wind chimes in the distance. Then we started to lift her up and drop her down. Lift up and drop down.

In less than a minute she started to sob almost uncontrollably. At this moment, while the three men held her body, I bent over her and hugged her deeply and strongly. I sensed that she had tremendous hurt and anger blocking in her abdomen and I took my hand and symbolically massaged it, withdrew it from her body, and cast it to the winds. At some deep level, we connected as eternal womanhood.

As the men cradled her and rocked her and I bent over her, her tears flowed. The rest of the group formed a quiet circle holding hands. Some of the men had tears in their eyes and the women had tenderness and compassion. At the close of this ritual, the entire group came and put their hands on Donna's body to give her the complete flow of their love. All of this took place in less than 15 minutes. Moments afterwards, Donna was on her feet running within the group and demonstrating one of the tempos.

Summary

In this chapter I have tried to explore the importance of alignment, strength and flexibility work, and show some of the tools, systems and healing techniques readily available to help you on your path toward fitness and awareness. You are only as healthy as your spine is aligned and flexible. And your feelings and sensations will increase in depth and magnitude as you include a flexibility program of 20 to 40 or more minutes a day in your schedule and three 30-minute sessions per week of strength training. Not only will you avoid and prevent the possibility of injury, you will start to play the upper edge of your fullest potential as a *human being*.

Prelude to
Men in Training:
Freeing the Hunter

Awakening the Heroic

I would say the common entry point for my work with men has to do with inspiration: the feeling that there is another way, a vitalistic approach to lifestyle that somehow makes sense intellectually and emotionally. But I have found that a mere intellectual appeal doesn't touch the heart. The ignition switch is the emotions and the feelings. And so with men, particularly, I always try to awaken feelings of joy, reverence, transcendence, inspiration, and to spark a sense of the heroic destiny which is often dormant in their consciousness. Unless you awaken the hero in a man, his training program can get very flat and monotonous.

One of my students told me of having his car locked in a city parking lot overnight. It was seven miles from his home. The next day he decided to use his training for a very practical application, running to get his car. He talked about what a beautiful and exciting experience it was. "I didn't exactly know the way to the parking lot, but I could spot certain buildings in the city and I used them to get my bearings. At one point I had to run up an expressway ramp. I had only about 12 inches of concrete on which to run. Cars were whizzing past me at 50 to 60 miles per hour. At another point, I had to run over a walkway that crossed a large river. I was running on an iron mesh overpass and I could look down through it to the water about 50 feet and see my reflection. In the city, I ran past a building with mirror walls and could watch myself run."

I said to Bill, "When you ran to get your car, you were protecting your family, you were braving the winds, the traffic, the unknown. You were like the hunter out there and that beautiful power that was being awakened in you was the hero, not the conquering hero but the hero of real inner power." This is the type of feeling I try to arouse in the men that I coach.

177

Chapter Eight:
Men in Training:
Freeing the Hunter

Men have paid a terrible price for their preeminent position in the business and professional world. Nowhere is this more evident than in a typical man's approach to running. All the logical, analytical, compulsive, competitive, driving forces surface when most men decide to get fit through running.

My goal in training men is not to diminish the heroic, the hunter, instinct in men but rather to free them to express this instinct as a loving human being rather than the cold, analytic, calculating, compulsive being that is often manifested.

Brotherhood vs. Narcissism

Most of the men I work with have had very few relationships with other men that are not hierarchical, where power, money, competition, manipulation, and judgment rule. There is always the expectation that the other man is somehow trying to subtly maneuver them. Really good corporate executives are excellent subtle manipulators. Deep in their psyches is a fear of expressing feelings, a fear that such expression will reveal their weaknesses which will then allow others to manipulate and dominate them. There is a fear of not measuring up to the competitive standards of other men. From my experience, I would say that most men are very lucky if they have one or two close male friends in relationships uncontaminated by these variables. The fact that a man doesn't have clear brotherhood with another man means that there is a lack of authenticity in his emotional responses. And there's always a delayed emotional response that occurs when you have to calculate your behavior by external variables based on power, competition, and manipulation. The net result is some form of stress.

So with men, one of the most beautiful things that can happen in their physical training program is they develop training buddies. A good example is the following which happened in one of my weekend workshops.

The Brotherhood of Hunters

The park in which we were doing our workouts was about a mile and a half from the Yoga Center where we gathered in the morning for preliminaries and at lunch for a light meal. The group in the workshop was widely varied in both physical condition and running experience. There were four men in the workshop just over 40 who were all serious runners and who almost immediately made contact with each other at a deep emotional level.

I first noticed them as a group after our first morning of training. Everyone was going back to the Yoga Center to have lunch. Most of us decided to walk back over. We were pairs and triplets, talking about things that had happened during the morning. But these four men, with a minimum of talk, had banded together and were running over the hill in the park toward the exit that led to the Yoga Center. Frank tells how the four came together and became training partners in a way that is totally different from most male associations in physical training.

> Bob and I had run together that morning before the workshop. I was staying at his house and we got started about 6:30 a.m. It was a gorgeous day. We ran to the park where the workshop was to be held. It was mostly rolling hills, with some beautiful flower beds, magnificent wooded areas, and dirt trails, some covered with wood shavings.
>
> There was something different about how Bob and I were running. We had both previously been exposed to Dyveke's training methods and this immediately dissipated any feeling of competition. Bob was used to running faster over shorter distances than I, but we accommodated our styles to each other. He ran just a shade slower than he usually did and I ran just a shade faster. There was absolutely no feeling that one of us was trying to "show up" the other by setting a faster than normal pace. Since it was Bob's trail, I stayed slightly behind and let him introduce me to his running world.
>
> We could easily pass the "talk test" so discussed in all the literature on running. The test specifies that most of your jogging be done at a pace that would allow you to carry on a conversation with a running partner. We were breathing easily, discussing how we usually ran alone, what winter had done to our training, how we had integrated the different running gaits and visualization techniques that Dyveke teaches into our training, and how that approach had changed our training from drudgery to fun. We also talked about how the training program we were putting together was for the rest of our lives and that we could afford to be pa-

tient with ourselves by taking days off from training and taking time to get advice and help for injuries instead of masochistically training through them.

Several times my mind flashed back to my running trails. And I would imagine Bob visiting me someday and my being able to show him my trails. This was a spiritual experience; having another person share his trail in a very loving, open way. I could imagine Bob getting up on a cold winter morning, running in here alone, passing familiar trees, rocks, and bushes that had long since become as friends. And, mostly without words, he was introducing me to these friends. My experiences in my own running world made it possible for me to understand what was happening.

From time to time we would see someone running toward us and we would all exchange "Good mornings." Bob would turn around and run backwards, or sideways, or break into an asymmetric gait. Sometimes I would follow and sometimes I would just continue in the gait I was running, deep into some visualization. We reached an area with small bushes separated by enough space for us to run in and out, around and through in a playful way. I got so involved that I fell behind Bob, who was moving to another area. But there was no hassle. When I was satisfied with my experience, I went off in the direction of Bob, who was running a large circular holding pattern, undoubtedly in the midst of some visualization of his own, as he waited for me. Then it was up some stone steps to a higher level and off down a path by a stream.

It's amazing the qualitative difference in the way one gets to know an area when it can be experienced from a relaxed running gait. There is no comparison when seeing it from a car, or even walking through it. There is something about running with awareness, as Dyveke teaches it, that lets one really *see* what is there. The usual interfering chatter in the mind is calmed and the environment can just come in, uncontaminated by the usual random commentary.

Bob and I got back to his house much later than we had planned. We had gotten involved in nature and in each other. We had spent time discussing our amazingly parallel experiences, both going through painful separations with our wives that were certain to lead to divorce. Now we were a little pushed for time. "Why don't we shower together?" Bob asked. I guess this would mean nothing to jocks who are used to locker room togetherness, but I hadn't showered communally with other men since I was in college. Over the years, a certain decorum had built up, a certain formality, a certain desire for privacy.

But all of a sudden, I felt a sense of brotherhood with Bob. We had just shared one of the most precious things two men could share, a run without competition through *his* trail. We had hugged each other very unselfconsciously at the end of the run. It wasn't the awkward sort of thing that sometimes happens between men but was our way of saying how close we felt. And now I was saying, "Hey, that's a great idea." Again, no self-consciousness. We undressed, went into the bathroom, got the shower going, talked about some books on Zen meditation. We both stood in the big bathtub, soaped ourselves, and took turns under the shower.

It is a first step for both of us in regaining some of the feelings of camaraderie that we left behind when we graduated from the relaxed world of the locker room and moved into the more formal world of our professions. But there was a difference in our new locker room. I wasn't trying to beat Bob out for the forward slot on the basketball team. He wasn't making fun of my clumsiness on the court. There was no class consciousness here. We were two equals trying to alter our lifestyles so that we could live more effectively in the New Age that is close at hand.

And yet, there was nothing to cast any doubt on our essential maleness. We had not even come close to surrendering the hunter instinct that is in us. We just had it in clearer perspective. The hunt isn't the end in and of itself. We can afford to be vulnerable, yet we know our strength and we can stand toe to toe physically or mentally with anyone.

This hunter instinct came out in our run from the park to the Yoga Center for lunch that day. We were joined by Jim, a lawyer who has practiced Zen for several years, who wants very much to run a marathon, who has gone through the divorce that Bob and I face, and has managed to put his life together with a new mate. And Brian. Brian has never been married. He is a career military officer who has been doing a lot of running and is in good physical condition. But in Brian there is none of the machismo that one often sees in military men. And that same deep strength that Bob and I have is in both Brian and Jim. You know that they could put up a tough fight. All four of us could, but we don't have to make a show of it.

Jim sets the pace as we leave the park. It is a good bit faster than I'm used to running, but I have laid the base of long, slow distance running and even with my morning run and a half day of the workshop in my body, I have plenty to spare. Up the steep, grass-covered hill. Down the other side and through a little valley, over a grassy trail, and finally to the stone fence that separates the park from the rest of the world. We slow at the fence and hop up and over.

Now we are on concrete. We are fired up from the workshop. We've spent the morning in a beautiful relaxed state first working on a sunstar visualization and then, while in a relaxed state, going through a long Feldenkrais exercise series. Then, maintaining our soft focus, we ran the shake-up and did almost an hour of interval training.

The four of us, who have laid the physical base, now want to extend ourselves. We are ready for the hunt. There is no feeling of competition between us, but there is the common prey. We are bonded. We will pool our energy. We will pursue our common goal. Our bodies are ready. We are oblivious of the rest of the world. We aren't mere men running down a Toronto street, we are hunters. Our spears are in our right hands. The animal in front of us is swift and cunning. It will try to exhaust us. But we will not be deterred. We have learned our lessons well. We keep our feet low, we take in oxygen and blow it out, making room for more. Our hands, arms, and shoulders are relaxed. But we are moving fast.

Jim is our leader. As we follow him, his presence pulls us along with him. We are all visualizing. The four are as one. No longer four, no longer men, no longer in Toronto, we are an energy system. It is not a race against each other. No interpersonal competition. But at the same time, we are giving all we have, 100 per cent. We will spare no effort. No machochism, no ego. A brotherhood. What foe could challenge us today? We will protect our women and our children. We will be living examples for our young men. We will make the kill, not because we like to kill but because the universe has made us hunters. Nothing can keep us from the prey. We are brothers.

Isn't this what they'd like to teach us in phys ed classes and in organized sports? Isn't this what we'd like them to teach our children? The hunter instinct in a man doesn't have to be eradicated. Teach him to become vulnerable without losing his instinct to be heroic, his instinct to be the protector. Teach him compassion, teach him to tap the intuitive knowledge within, help him rediscover beauty and tenderness while maintaining that insuperable will, that forceful drive that no wall can contain. The man of men. The vulnerable hunter.

I remember that day, looking at these four men running with the group and obviously in much better condition than the others. I watched the tenderness and compassion that came through as the men were doing sensing and innerspace work. I watched as they developed a sense of closeness and brotherhood as training buddies.

As a woman coach I try, more than anything, to awaken in the psyche of men in training a spontaneity and connection to their feelings. I have them record emotional explosions, dreams, free-flowing streams of consciousness in journals. It can have a very profound effect their personal relationships with everyone they meet. And if their physical training is *not* having that effect on their lives, then I feel that my work as a woman coach is not effective.

It is extremely important for a man beginning a physical training program to understand that all the setbacks, all the hardships, all the injuries, all the stupid things that he can do to his body are lessons to learn about self-transformation. There is often an incredible underlying guilt if anything goes wrong in his body. He assumes he is at fault. He wonders what he has to blame himself for. And the self-reproach, self-criticism and self-condemnation eats away at his self-love. If that cycle gets started, it only strengthens his need to dominate. So he has to examine his life, his network of interpersonal relations, his methods of communications. He must ask how much of his life is based on narcissism and self-preoccupation, how much is other-directed, in the sense of letting everyone else's needs determine his priorities, and how to balance his energy with concern for social and humanitarian issues.

Often I meet a narcissistic, self-centered male who thinks the whole world revolves around his sport. As the feminine principle begins to come into his consciousness, and the principles of a vitalistic training program start to permeate his life, and he gets feedback, he will slowly start to incorporate that sense of the hero into his life.

Sensitive, Self-doubting Men

There is another type of man, the sensitive, self-doubting man who questions his sexual potency, who is a little frustrated in his relationship with

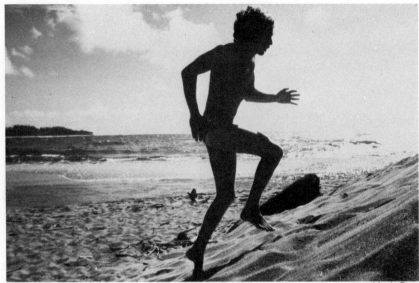

Marcia Cross

women, and maybe has a not-too-interesting job. After a period of long, slow distance training, I usually put him on very intensive interval training in which he will have explosions and develop a sense of tremendous power.

Or I'll surprise him after a very nurturing period of running on a mountain or around a track. As I am touching his back and visualizing light streamers and fountains and seed thoughts, all very sensitive things, I'll say very casually, "Now I'd like you to do some very fast intervals. You stay at my left shoulder." I'll push him right up to his limits when he's ready to handle it. But I treat it offhandedly. I'll back away and not say anything, just give him an experience, a fantastic breakthrough in his training, without putting any concept around it. In essence I'm helping him experience the instant feedback of masculinity as an athlete that he's never really felt. Through his body he has touched the heroic.

The Hard-Driving Executive

At the other end of the spectrum is the extremely disciplined, hard-driving, one-focused type A, compulsive man, who has a phenomenally busy schedule with too many demands. I always use long slow distance training with such a person to bring about a meditative, stress-reducing, nonjudgmental attitude. With that type of man it is extremely important to get the stream of consciousness journals going. I, as the coach, need concrete feedback in writing of what he understands to be happening in his consciousness. And he needs to be able to go back and read it. This kind of man needs concrete reinforcement and feedback. And this helps to siphon off the linear left-brain processes through which he usually operates. A man will be willing to put down stop watches and log books if he has some substitute for them.

You don't strip away the process that gives a man his power. Rather, you add a process that awakens the feminine principle already present. I would say if I had to make certain generalizations that it is totally, completely astounding to me how little it takes to awaken these natural instincts in the male psyche. I often stand back in awe and reverence. Sometimes it takes no more than a consultation, one or two training sessions, and a few phone calls. On other occasions, it's somebody attending a workshop that I don't see again for three to six months to a year. Then I may get a letter, phone call, or bump into them on the street. Many of my clients with whom I have had long-term one-, two- or three-year relationships have ended up working with me to plan or build some project. They end up wanting to be an assistant. They have an avocation. They want to be a New Age coach.

Why Men Come to Me

I become the coach of the men who come to me for a variety of reasons. First, there is stress and loss of meaning in their lives. Second, the system they are using is either causing or aggravating some dormant injury and not allowing them to maintain their training program. Third is a kind of hopelessness and helplessness about getting their lives reorganized in a holistic way. They really need counseling and guidance for those phases.

I have seen so many types of men. Tom is a high executive with the Department of Health, Education and Welfare who has incredible job stress, family problems and ideological conflict. His running has changed his sedentary lifestyle and altered his professional outlook. He wants bureaucracy to be responsive to human needs and his own life to reflect tenderness, openess, authenticity. He's in transition at all levels.

Bill is a sensitive New Age man. His feelings have been awakened. He is very aware, into yoga, Zen, philosphy. He wants to get into a training program that will awaken a flame in his masculine instinct. But he wants to do it in a way that won't destroy the sensitivity that he has worked so hard to develop.

Jerry is an outstanding athlete in his early thirties, handsome, sensitive, good at business but wants his sports training time to be approached less compulsively. He's fearful of longstanding injuries and needs guidance in stabilizing his training program to avoid continually reinjuring his body. He wants to be more in touch with feelings, expressing emotions honestly. He's willing to devote tremendous discipline to work on himself.

John, a 50-year-old psychiatrist, has a highly developed consciousness. He is a very aware, sensitive person, deeply into all the lore of the human potential movement and holistic health. But he is also overworked, overburdened, overpeopled, and never takes any time for himself.

Bob, a 50-year-old athlete, has had cataclysmic injuries but has a passion for team sports. As coach of a team, he had the vision to carry everything he learned from me to the team. But his life is characterized by high stress. He is a hard-driving, type A personality with an overachieving syndrome.

Larry, is an over-40 executive who has never really had a chance to get in touch with his body. He has been the subject of too many demands for too many years, and has suddenly reached a tilt point. He has an ulcer. There is emotional stress in his family. Mainly there is the ennui; life no longer has any meaning. He is searching for spiritual awakening and love of self, love of body, love of humanity.

Matthew is a 30-year-old who is *making it* professionally. His family and love relationship is basically working. He is dabbling in a lot of different sports. He's not sick or injured but isn't quite turned on. Life is a little bit flat.

Jim is a world-class competitive athete. He is highly trained, highly competitive, highly skilled, extremely disciplined, but has huge missing links in his understanding of the holistic health approach to training.

And then there is Ralph. He is in his late forties. He has had a heart attack. He is really frightened and uses repression, denial, and escapism to avoid fear. But there also is an overtone of hopelessness, helplessness, and semi-depression.

I suspect that deep in the psyches of most men not in good physical shape is a great sense of loss. It's not sadness or self-condemnation, it's more subtle. It's very similar to a child who's never had an opportunity to play and who exhibits a certain solemnity. I would say that with men in training, the singular most important variable is to *adopt a playful attitude*, because out of playfulness comes joy, self-transcendence, and quiet moments of inner awakening. Out of a sense of play also comes the relinquishment of compulsive, competitive patterns. Every time I help a man develop a lifestyle training program, it is based on some kind of cardiovascular conditioning such as running, swimming, or biking. But I also try to help him move over into some kind of game: tennis, racquet ball, rugby.

Bill: Training in Ignorance

Bill is a perfect example of how many men start a type of training program that is almost guaranteed doom in a short time. Bill is an engineer who has gone into business with one of his former professors. He is 33 years old and beginning to chafe under the structure that has evolved with his business partner. Bill is growing as an individual but still feels somewhat like a glorified graduate student. When he goes to the office in the morning, a pain erupts in his right side as he reaches for the door. He is not really aware of it on a conscious level but it manifests itself in an overall feeling that something is wrong.

Bill works a nine- to ten-hour day and then goes home, exhausted, to have a meal with his wife and their two small children. Then he watches a little television and reads the paper. Once or twice a week, he and his wife go out. Bill keeps seeing articles about physical fitness. He keeps telling himself that he doesn't have time. About a year ago, Bill met a fellow engineer whom he came to respect and admire. The friend was a runner and the topic kept coming up whenever they were together.

One day, it all gelled for Bill: the articles, his memories of games and sports when he was a chlld, what his friend had said. It came together and Bill decided it was time to do something about his physical condition. His friend had pointed out the need to have good shoes, so Bill went to a well-known men's shoe store and bought an expensive pair of running shoes. There were several models but the sales clerk didn't seem to know much about running shoes. Bill figured that he couldn't go wrong getting the most expensive pair. They felt a little tight but the clerk said they would loosen up.

The next step was to get his car out and measure off a course around the streets near his home so that he would know exactly how far he ran each time. Bill knew nothing about stretching, body alignment, strength training, or nutrition. But he did know how to put one foot in front of the other and he figured that that was a good way to start. He remembered from school that he needed some kind of warmup. There was a very steep hill near his house and Bill figured that a good warmup would be to run up and down this hill several times before beginning his main run on the more level course that he had charted. So he drove up and down the hill to get the mileage.

Bill decided to be very logical about the whole process. He knew that there are individual differences among people and he figured that he should start out at his own rate and try to shave time off each workout.

It was mid-March when Bill started. He would come home at night, eat a big steak, a huge plate of spaghetti, or a pizza with the family. Then he'd sit around and read the paper. Finally, about 9:00, he would put on two pairs of dungarees, two shirts, gloves, a ski hat, and his new jogging shoes. He would jump up, bolt out the door, pause until the second hand on his watch was straight up, and take off full speed down the steep hill. Then he would struggle for all he was worth back up to the top. Three round trips and he was ready to start his main run.

He would get another time check and tear down the street, the stop watch clicking away the seconds, his feet pounding on the concrete pavement of the street. Shoulders high and tight. Fists clenched. Cold air searing his throat. A stitch in the right side. The half-mile mark. A glance at the stop watch. "Dammit. I'm ten seconds off tonight. Christ, I can't catch my breath. It was so easy last night." The pain in the side is worse. Then the pain in the left knee, feeling almost as though it were out of joint. Gasping for breath. "All this pain is a good sign. It means I'm really getting a good workout tonight."

During the run, he would be cloaked in a cloud of gloom. This was his running night. It seemed like no time since he was out here before. "Why do I have to be so conscious when I'm running? It's so hard. There is no enjoyment. It's like taking a horrible-tasting medicine that you know will help but that seems nearly as bad as the ailment."

As he ran, Bill would spend most of his time thinking about how hard running is, how lonely. He would feel a certain amount of self-righteousness; all those other people sitting around watching tv. "By God, when they start having heart attacks, they'll wish they had done something about it." At every mile, Bill would check his watch and madly start subtracting current time from starting time or last mile time to find out his time for this mile. It was a little discouraging. Bill knew about four minute miles. And of course he realized that he could never reach that level. But still, a ten minute mile seemed pretty slow. And what's more, it was not improving all that much from night to night. Bill could fantasize about being an athlete, but these times would be laughable in any competition he could imagine.

Then there were the dogs, the kids, the cars. There is one spot at which he'd always get startled. A big black dog would give a mighty bark, lunge out toward him, only to be snapped back by a chain. Bill would knot up his forehead, feel a little squirt of adreneline, curse lightly, and keep pounding out his constant beat on the pavement. And it always seemed that when his energy was at its lowest he'd meet a bunch of kids. "There goes the bionic man." He know he was going slow but this was ridiculous. Then there was always the car stopped at an intersection that would blast out just as Bill got three-quarters of the way past it. So many times he pushed his left hand against the fender of the accelerating car to steady himself.

And then there were the other joggers. He'd hear footsteps behind him and recognize the sound of another jogger overtaking him, then passing and, too quickly, leaving him behind. At such points, he would try to speed up, try to at least maintain the speed of the runner now opening a large gap between them. Finally, he would have to slack off to a pace he could maintain.

At the end of the run, he would check his watch for the time of his last mile, rush into the house, fall down on the couch exhausted, and watch tv for a while. Then he would struggle up, have a coke and some cookies or cake, and finally make it to the shower.

His running was erratic. Sometimes he would run for eight or nine days in a row. Then he would miss four or five. Then he'd run two or three times in a row and miss six or seven. He had a lot of blisters. But worse, he began to feel some pain in his knees. Then he started to notice a swelling in his right knee. It became bigger but Bill said, "A little pain can't stop me." He started having trouble walking. But regardless, every time he ran he would warm-up by pounding down the 45-degree hill on hard pavement.

It finally got to the point where he just couldn't run anymore. The pain was too much. "I'll let it rest for a few weeks and then get started again." His running shoes and time and distance logbook were put aside, then packed away and finally thrown out. Bill would try to play basketball with his friends once in a while but in 15 or 20 minutes his knees would start swelling. "I'd love to run or play basketball, but I've ruined my knees." That did help salve his conscience.

Where Did Bill Go Wrong?

Bill had an admirable goal, forestalling a heart attack. But he needed a coach at that point. The attrition rate for those beginning physical fitness programs is about 70 percent. This is not surprising to anyone who knows about training. Getting started in a training program sounds as if it should be so simple. Get a pair of shoes and start running. After all, nothing is more natural than running.

It can be simple and easy if you know what you're doing. But I have spent years distilling information about running techniques, weight training, nutrition, body therapies, approaches to flexibility, visualizations. I can spend two hours with a person and set up a Lifestyle Training Program that will be appropriate and that he will be able to follow for the rest of his life. But this is because I know what to look for. I have helped literally hundreds avoid back operations. By some simple recommendations concerning body alignment, I have helped many men lay a training base on a properly aligned body and thus avoid possible serious injury. Simple programs for achieving deep relaxation and the use of visualizations have helped many men turn training into a pleasurable, rewarding experience.

Bill's first and probably biggest mistake was that he didn't set up his physical training program as part of an overall Lifestyle Training Program. He tried to fit it in with his present lifestyle and it wasn't very compatible. He did nothing about his nutrition. He applied a great deal of stress to his body but did nothing to replace the nutrients he was using. His regular diet might have gotten him through a nonphysical existence, but as soon as he started to live the life of an athlete, he needed an athlete's nutritional program.

Bill needed to see himself as an *athlete in training*. There is something justifiably heroic about such a view. It puts everything in a new perspective. "I have to watch what I'm eating because I'm an *athlete in training*.. "I need to take my vitamin and mineral supplements because I'm an *athlete in train-*

ing. "I need to do a proper warmup and cooldown procedure because I'm an *athlete in training*. "I need to take one day off per week from my training schedule because I'm an *athlete in training*. You can see that the proper approach to training demands a whole new way of looking at life.

This process can be greatly facilitated with a coach. If I could work with each of you personally, I could cut months and maybe years off the process. But there aren't enough coaches to go around, so I'm using this book as one substitute. You won't progress as fast as you would if you could work directly with me. You will have to take more responsibility for yourself and your training program. And yet, by carefully studying the material in this book, you can benefit from my years of study and prevent needless injury and agony in your training.

For example, Bill didn't realize that his right foot was slightly turned out with the result that the thousands of pounds of additional pressure he was putting on his right knee during running was being applied at an unnatural angle.

Bill realized that proper shoes are the most important part of a runner's gear. But he didn't know the proper approach to purchasing them. It is essential to buy shoes from a store with personnel who know something about running. Many runners are putting needless blisters on their feet, losing toenails, bruising bones because they, like Bill, have confused the most expensive shoe with the best fitting shoe.

In another area, Bill knew nothing about proper warmup. Instead of doing stretches that would prepare his legs and body for the stress to be applied during running, Bill was banging up his knees with an all-out downhill run. He took the aching in his body on the day after a run as a sign that he had gotten some benefit out of the run.

And, of course, Bill had no idea of how to utilize his most valuable ally, his mind, in his physical training. Pain, negativity, and ego accompanied him on every run when he could have been experiencing transcendent moments of bliss. In the following sections, I am going to deal with some of the problems that men face in training. Most of these problems arise from a very admirable trait found in most men, an ability to be one-pointed, focused, to surmount all obstacles. But in most men, this aspect is out of control and needs to be harnessed, not done away with but harnessed.

I advised Bill to leave his stopwatch at home when he was running and to start a program of long slow distance training. Before a run, he would read a short poem, listen to a piece of music, or read a passage from some inspirational book. On the run itself, he would let his mind be still and allow the sights and sounds of nature to enter his consciousness. He wouldn't carry on a running description of what he saw, but would just experience it. He would find a favorite tree and go around it twice on each run. He would run in a playful manner: sometimes backwards, sometimes sideways, sometimes fast, sometimes slow. Through this series of rituals, Bill began to feel that he was getting in touch with his inner self and with the outer world of nature. He began to be inspired by the beauty his soul was touching every day. Bill has had little trouble keeping his training program going since he became more skillful in using his will.

Men and Lifestyle Assessment

Most men tend to want to "get on with it." They often begin a training program with either a rather nebulous, general goal or a rather specific, narrow goal: wanting to feel better, wanting to look better, wanting to show those around them that they aren't washed up physically, wanting to avoid a heart attack, wanting to set an example for their children. And it is typical that the stimulus to get started comes from some newspaper, magazine article, book, from seeing an old friend who is going downhill, or meeting someone his own age who is in much better condition.

But most of the time there is no period of self-assessment with an attempt to fit the physical training into an improved overall lifestyle. This is unfortunate because a training approach that is not an integral part of one's lifestyle is almost certain to fail. A typical male reaction when reading this book would be to pass lightly over Chapter Two on self-assessment and go straight to the Chapter Four on moving. If you did that, I urge you to retrace your steps and carefully go through Chapter Two. Follow the procedures to the letter and try to ascertain what it is you want out of life. The physical training portion of your Lifestyle Fitness Program should be based on your answer to this question, not on some general goal such as feeling better or something very specific such as wanting to trim two inches off your waistline.

I have helped many men start Lifestyle Training Programs that they have been able to maintain in the face of hectic schedules and difficult family situations. Without exception, all of these programs have started with an individual consultation which began by getting the person into a deeply relaxed state and continued with a deep exploration of where the person is with regard to his family, work and friends, and where he would like to be. I always help him grapple with the question of what life would be like for him if he could have his wildest dream.

It is only after we have dealt satisfactorily with these questions and arrived at a goal, that it makes sense to begin designating the physical training portion of his Lifestyle Training Program. And the approach is not always running. For some men, swimming is a better approach to endurance because of weather conditions, time factors, personal preference. It is important to see a Lifestyle Training Program as encompassing all aspects of one's life and as lasting for the rest of one's life. It is not just trimming two inches off the middle but keeping the two inches off. That is a lifetime proposition.

It is also important that any training program be realistic. You might want to set up a running program that will include five miles a day. But you might be too busy to make this a realistic goal. If you carefully assess your current lifestyle, you may be able to find areas that you can adjust so that you can get in the five miles. But after careful study, you may not be able to find enough time under current conditions. In the latter case, you will need to adjust your expectations to maybe four miles per day or five miles four times per week. If you try to crowd in too much, you will only end up slighting some other area and feeling guilty about it, or finally giving up your whole running program because you can't meet the goal you have set.

The point of a training program is to get your body working efficiently so that you have more energy to enjoy life and so that your body is strong, flexible, and durable enough to participate more fully in life: dance, hike, canoe, swim. Any fitness program should be pointed toward this end. For most people, the training program itself should not be the end but rather the means to a much fuller end.

Men and Flexibility Training

Most men are looking for quick results, some tangible differences that their training is producing. Endurance and strength training both offer this kind of immediate feedback in ways that men can relate to. For example, being able to steadily increase the distance that one is running provides evidence that something is happening in training. The same is true in strength training where one is able to add more weight to each exercise as the weeks of training go by. In running, the person begins to feel better, more alive and has more energy. In strength training, he can see his muscles begin to tone up and get larger.

For many men, the results don't necessarily have to be pleasant. The feeling of physical pain that is often present in untrained running, the burning sensation in muscles when an impossibly heavy weight is being wrestled with in strength training, the feeling of total exhaustion, the aching muscles after a hard workout, are often taken as signs that the training is working. If it's producing pain and exhaustion, it must be doing some good.

This kind of attitude, prevalent in men, often leads to a lot of skepticism and disinterest when it comes to flexibility and innerspace training. There is a similar problem with nutrition, but it often stems from actual rather than imagined inconveniences.

I talked to Tim quite a bit about flexibility. He runs 25 to 30 miles and works out with weights several hours per week. We talked often about flexibility and how it was very important for him to do stretches to minimize the chance of injury when running. We did quite a few of them in his individual training sessions. But I could tell that he was not very enthusiastic about flexibility.

"It's so hard for me to see how these exercises are helping me. We lie down on the ground and move into some position which puts a strain on some muscle set. Then we hold it for a few seconds and go to a new position. We aren't working the muscles back and forth at all. There is no perspiration. My heart isn't beating much faster than if I were reading a book. And there are so many positions. I've tried to follow the directions in a book but it's so complicated and I never know if I'm doing it right. When I run, it's obvious that something is happening. When I lift weights, it's obvious that something is happening. But when I'm stretching, it isn't obvious that *anything* is happening. Wouldn't I be better off spending that time running? I could just run very slowly for the first half mile and that should warm me up."

One morning, several weeks later, Tim called me and said, excitedly, "Something clicked in me this morning. I ran day before yesterday and my legs ached all night. I woke up one time and remembered what you had told me about the importance of doing at least a five-minute cooldown after a run followed by a few basic stretches. Then next morning, I saw an article in the paper on jogging. The author said that without a proper cooldown period, blood pools in your legs and lactic acid is not cleared and that it's the lactic acid that's responsible for most of the muscle aches you get the day after exercise."

Tim was now psychologically ready for flexibility work. I reminded him of four basic stretches that we had worked on: one for the calves, one for the hamstring, one for the quadriceps, and one for the adductors. "Do those before you run and after you run and see how your legs feel tonight."

Tim called me the next day. "I did these stretches before I ran. At the end of my run I walked for five minutes versus my usual two and then I did the stretches again. I can't tell you what a difference I feel in my legs. There was none of the aching last night that I usually experience, none of the stiffness in my legs that I usually feel if I sit around for an hour or so after running. I feel as if my training has made a quantum leap."

Men and Weight Training

Most men have tried some weight training at one time or another. But they usually come to it with a rather macho approach. A man training by himself may get a set of weights with an instruction booklet. His first instinct is to go too fast. If the booklet says ten repetitions with ten pounds, he will try 15 repetitions with 15 pounds. And he will struggle for all he is worth to get through the repetitions. He will, in general, ignore form, and do the repetitions some way, thinking that the important thing is to somehow get the weights there and back when actually the form is a critical component.

What he fails to appreciate is that it's important to be able to go through the whole recommended movement in the specified way. This means using a weight that enables him to do the repetitions the prescribed way. A weight that hinders this, hinders his progress.

There is even more of a temptation to use weights that are too heavy when working in a group atmosphere such as a gym. After all, there are other men around who are lifting much heavier weights. And it's hard to admit that you can't do as much as any other male. Few men can resist this temptation, and many retard their training by proceeding with such an attitude.

I'll never forget one of my first visits to a Nautilus gym. Nautilus is a weight training system that uses scientifically designed machines to apply a variable force to the muscles so that each portion gets the amount of weight it can handle. As I talked to one of the owners, I heard an awful gasping, groaning, straining noise. It sounded a lot like someone going through a bioenergetics exercise to get out anger but somehow holding back.

I looked up and saw the 45-year-old man in a life-and-death struggle with the rowing machine. Instead of moving through a repetition smoothly but with effort, he was exerting extreme effort and stopping and starting through the movement. The perspiration was flowing down his beet-red face, veins bulging out. It was obvious he didn't understand the principles involved in strength training. He was operating on a typical male principle, that if it's hard enough and painful enough, it must be working.

This wasn't my only experience of this type. It almost never fails when I'm doing a Nautilus workout that at least one other person will be struggling with weights too heavy for his particular stage of development. But he will be giving it his all, with awful gasps and moans, completely oblivious of how he is hindering his training. Bob, one of the owners of this Nautilus franchise, says, "There are a lot of guys who approach their weight training this way. They just won't listen to us."

Even the more *enlightened* men aren't exempt from these tendencies. Joe tells of this experience.

> When I first started my Nautilus training, I was well aware of the basic principles involved: doing a given number of repetitions, eight to 12, at a weight that would leave you unable to do another repetition after the twelfth one. I have a rather large frame but am actually somewhat weak in my upper body. My Nautilus instructor recommended some starting weights. My fiancé, who had already worked out at Nautilus several times, expressed amazement at out how much weight I could handle. These weights actually felt too heavy to me but I struggled through with them. The instructor said I should increase each by five pounds at each workout.
>
> I admit that the words of my fiancé had inflated my ego and it was hard for me to admit that I had too much weight. Over the next few sessions, I strayed from the Nautilus principles several times in order to impress my fiancé and my Nautilus instructor. It wasn't easy to admit my weights

were too heavy. I'd see the weights being used by those in front of me and feel envious when their weight for that particular machine was heavier than mine. Deep down inside I knew what I should do, but I couldn't bring myself to do it.

Finally, one day I walked in for my workout and said to myself, "That's enough of this nonsense. I'm going to find the right weight for me for each of these damn machines and stay with it until I can do the right number of repetitions with the proper form. Then and only then will I increase the weight." I looked at my progress card. For a couple of the machines, the correct weight was the one I was using now. I had started with 70 pounds on the leg machine and had now increased it to 90 pounds. And I was making the recommended number of repetitions with good form. But for most of the other machines, I had to drop the weight down. In some cases, I had to go back to my starting weight.

Over the next few sessions, I increased my weight on a couple of machines, but on the others, I had to stay at the same weight. I now feel much better psychologically. I know that eventually I'll get my weights up to a level that will impress both my fiancé and instructor. But in the meantime, I have the satisfaction of knowing that I'm doing my training correctly. I'm not here to impress people but to build up my strength and tone up my body. I'm taking a longer view. I have time. But even when you know better, sometimes it's hard to keep your priorities straight.

Because of cultural conditioning and deep instinctual feelings, many men are prone to begin projects as if they were raging bulls, ready to charge over, around or through all obstacles, showing no patience. Such an approach can lead to serious injuries, and even if an injury doesn't result, it will make the training process so difficult and distasteful that the motivation to continue a training program will shrivel and eventually die.

One of my students tells how his compulsiveness tended to doom any attempts at training.

I used to periodically get interested in exercising. I would get a book that would really impress me and I'd start the program. But I wanted results, so I'd begin to increase my exercise time each day. If the book recommended five minutes of running in place, I'd find myself adding five minutes each day. It would finally result in taking more than an hour each day to complete my exercise. Then I'd miss a few days and try to start back where I'd left off instead of gradually working back up. It would either be too hard to do it or I would decide that it just wasn't worth it and scrap the whole thing.

Men need to learn to harness this extreme enthusiasm, and keep their training program within reason and on track. One of the best ways of doing this is to make sure that your physical training program is part of a total lifestyle approach. It must not be an isolated segment that bears only a tangential relationship to everything else. And it must be seen as part of a process that will be pursued for the rest of your life. That means taking the long view. The goal won't be reached tomorrow. It will take time, but there is time to take.

Men and Nutrition

The difficulty men have with nutrition is not that they fail to see its relevance, but that they often find it inconvenient to implement. If a man is part of a family unit not particularly concerned with nutrition, there will be problems. Men also have the problem of business lunches and dinners, and ordering lunch from the nearest hamburger emporium.

Tom tells how he came to an acceptable though not perfect solution.

I've gotten myself onto a Lifestyle Training Program but I still have to live in a world that for the most part isn't concerned with good health and nutrition. I have had to learn to compromise. I'm married and we have three children. My wife and kids sometimes think I'm a little weird, like when I get up at 5 a.m. to run. I want to bring some of the ideas of health and nutrition into my family but it is going to take time. We've been living the other way too long. So I've figured out a fairly good way to alter my own nutrition without causing undue hardship on the family.

We've never eaten breakfast together, so I use that meal to get the grains, nuts, and fruit that I have neglected in the past. I train early and make my own breakfast. Without too much trouble I can put on a hot cereal to cook while I bathing after my run. I top it with yogurt, fruit, and granola. It really gets my day off to a good start. About ten minutes after eating breakfast, I take my supplements. Sometimes the kids are up at breakfast: they have presweetened cereal, but several times they have joined me in eating some of my cereal. They even admitted that it's not bad. I have to watch myself and not become too pushy with them.

My next problem area is snacks during work. I used to get some coffee and doughnuts about 10:30 or so. Now I make it a practice to have some mixed nuts like brazil nuts, peanuts, almonds, pumpkin seeds along with raisins and dates in my desk. Instead of getting doughnuts, I get a handful of peanuts. I also try to remember to bring several pieces of fruit to the office with me each day, an orange, banana, apple, pear.

Then there's the whole business about lunch. I may have to take customers to lunch, or a group of us at the office will go out for lunch together. These lunches are very important and in the past I've found them very enjoyable. But it often does present a problem in terms of sticking with my new approach to nutrition. I don't want to be a spoilsport or killjoy. I want to set a good example without being obnoxious.

It's getting to where many restaurants have salad bars now, and when that is the case, I always get a big salad. It's a little harder when everyone wants to go to a fast food place. But you can't win them all. A hamburger now and then isn't going to be disastrous.

Dinner can also be a little tricky. My family is big on spaghetti, steak, and fried foods; all things that I really liked in the past but which I'm trying to minimize in my present diet. When we go out to a restaurant, which we do a couple of times a week, it isn't too hard. I usually get broiled fish, a baked potato, and a salad. And at home, we've made a compromise. At least one night a week, we have a meal that I cook. It's a model of nutrition, yet done in a subtle way. Thus there are three or four nights a week out of the seven that I feel I'm doing pretty well, nutritionally. The others . . . well, Rome wasn't built in a day.

I've always been a midnight snack person myself. I know that it isn't recommended. But at least my snack these days is an improvement over what I used to have. I used to end my day with a big slice of cake and a soft drink. Now I usually have some granola and yogurt. I find I'm growing somewhat addicted to it.

I don't always feel great about my solution. I'm the type who likes to go all the way when I'm doing something. But I don't live in a vacuum. Besides, I learned from seeing one of my friends approach the situation the wrong way. He got hooked on nutrition and began a campaign to get his family to shape up. He had been married twenty years and never said a word about nutrition before. It became a war of wills with him on one side and his wife and children on the other. They had some real battles. And then he alienated many of the people at his office with his constant harangue about coffee, soft drinks, doughnuts, pizza, ad nauseum. Of course he was right, but he went about it in such a way that he alienated everyone in sight and actually gave nutrition a bad name.

So I take the position that each person is responsible for his or her own nutrition. I'll try to set a good but reasonable example. I'll get my body in such great shape that people will be *asking me* how I did it. As I said, my approach isn't perfect but it is basically doing the job.

Men and Innerspace

Many men are so at home with the principle that if it's painful, if it's hard, if it's distasteful, it must be working, that they completely miss the chance to turn training into a transcendent experience. We've cited many instances already of men who have approached physical training with a new purpose. They've learned how to still their minds and allow the beauty of nature to come in unfiltered, to allow repressed feelings to come out, to allow the knowledge within to surface. In such a training approach, the physical part of the workout serves as a stimulus to elicit transcendent moments while the total experience results in physical benefits such as a strengthening of the cardiovascular system.

Men, in their hurry to get to the point, to get down to business, are prone to dismiss things like lifestyle assessment, flexibility, and visualization, not appreciating that these are not dispensible frills, but rather the lifeblood of a training program.

Innerspace is especially important to men who all too often live in a logical, analytical world, lacking in tenderness, compassion, beauty, intuition. It can be the first step in helping a man to reevaluate the place of these things in a full and complete lifestyle. Once a man begins running *not* to surpass yesterday's record but to touch the trees, grass and bushes in a favorite park, to feel the sun sink deeply into his pores, to smile at ducks, squirrels and birds on his trail, to commune with ancestors who moved over the same paths and those yet unborn who will run on this same trail, his life will take on a whole new quality. He will be unleashing the full force of his feminine energy to complement his already well-developed masculine energy. The vulnerable hunter: he will never again be willing to go back to his old way of living.

A Woman Coach

I find that one of the things the men I coach admire in me is that I play many sports well. Not only am I a long-distance runner, but I can do high diving, long-distance swimming, play tennis, ski, badminton, and even coach rugby players. There's a little bit of ego identification here; if she can do it, so can I. I never put it out that way but, at a subliminal level, men realize that there are not that many women who can step into the consciousness of a man. Maybe the reason I can understand the consciousness of the man so well is because I have played so many of these sports. I know their passions, fears, and breaking points.

Most men really appreciate the sensitivity of a woman with whom they can share their deepest fears, their anxieties about their bodies. I assume the collective role of all of the female energies they've come into contact with: their sister, their lover, their mother, their high priestess, their teacher, their psychologist, their goddess. And through watching their reactions as I assume these roles, I can determine the relationships of these roles to the psyche of a man. Men relate to me through all these different roles of the female principle. I find that the definition of *chameleon* fits me. There is an element of changeability. And this is where the artist in me is really drawn on to the fullest extent, because I operate not only at the analytical level, but also completely relate at the emotional level. I'm always looking at the full spectrum, the flow.

As a woman coach, it is important to adopt at the beginning both the feminine and masculine way of relating. I am very receptive when taking in data. I just listen, because with men timing is very important. They must feel satisfied that they have told *their* story *their* way. And they must feel satisfied that I, as a woman, have listened to it. I might wait an hour to say something that only takes 30 seconds.

My job is to paint a portrait of the *person that is possible*, though now lying dormant, within them. So I help them to imprint a different self-image from that they have currently. It often happens after asking, "What is your wildest dream?" It is very important to plug into their ego ideal, the people they admire, the dream they have about themselves, the person they used to be. Somehow there's the hunter instinct, the heroic, the sense of personal power that most men have. I have coached men in their forties who still deep down inside have professional athletes — baseball, basketball, football players — as ego ideals.

Somehow, being a woman coach who can meet a man at his power level also gives him permission to break down at the sensitivity level. It is not at all uncommon for a very proud, self-composed man to break down in tears at the end of the workshop, either in my arms, the arms of another woman in the workshop, or in the arms of another man, and feel absolutely comfortable, accepted and unembarrassed. I'm not surprised when this comes following a really intensive day of training where sensing and innerspace experiences are blended with opening up to nature and other people. Most men simply don't think about training the physical body and simultaneously looking at the variables that need to be considered, such as alignment, energy flow in the body called "chi" flow (see Chapter 10), toxicity, feelings.

Second, I'm utterly astounded at how little it takes. Because of the natural instinct and wisdom of the body, even the most compulsive, driving men see that these principles make sense, and they get immediate feedback. And they are "willing to try."

Third, I am also very surprised at the lack of chauvinism, even in some of the most up-tight conservative corporations where the only relationships men have had with women have been those in which men were dominant.

Fourth, the body is the temple of the spirit. The temple will never be complete for any man unless he is able to awaken the feminine principle that lies deep in his psyche.

Prelude to
Women in Training:
Reowning Your Power

"It's a very fortunate man indeed who can bring out the *Hetaera* in a woman!"

I looked into the clear, blue, Norwegian eyes of Jeanne Gibbs as she spoke. It was she who had become my *Hetaera* and had drawn me from Boston to her mountain retreat at Echo Lake, California. It had been revealed to me in meditation that I should come here to finish the chapter on women.

Jeanne continued, "There are four types of women. The Hetaera is the most celebrated, the most rewarded because she's the siren who calls forth the potential in man. From the earliest of times, men have depended on her. She rides the bow of the ship and guides the sailors. She calls them forth with her mystical qualities. The Hetaera woman helps the man to be all that he dare not be on his own.

"Men have created some of the greatest inventions in the world because women have had the capacity to make them feel ten feet tall. Men don't always feel ten feet tall. The Hetaera woman has helped to produce the progress of the world and has rarely gotten credit for it."

I felt that I was sitting at the feet of a very wise woman: athletic, a brilliant admininstrator, deeply into the mystical teaching of the esoteric traditions. My intuitions about coming here had been absolutely accurate.

"But, Dyveke, there are three other types of woman. There's the mother, the nurturer, the one who takes care of the family unit. She's the epitome of Eros, relatedness, the love energy of the world. The mother in women

201

must be brought forth because people hurt and need care: feeding, nurturing, protection. The mother has had a celebrated place throughout history.

"Then there's the Midean or the Mistrael, the wise old woman who is objective, has an essential knowingness, who can stand back and be wise and not be caught in trivia. She's the high priestess; prophetic, devotional, with an inner quietness and transcendence. She's in touch with the evolution of the soul. She has the devastating quality of *woman's intuition*."

Jeanne's eyes started to sparkle as she said, "And now, finally, women are again becoming the Amazon: strong, powerful, independent, and athletic. We're often Amazons whem we're young. We're into our bodies, independent. But now that's happening to women of all ages. That's part of the woman's movement. The Amazon spirit is saying, 'Hey, you men, I'm sick of calling you forth. I'm going to do my own thing in the world.' "

The resurgence of the Amazon energies is what women are bringing to sports. They're saying, "I've got to value myself, to take care of myself. I don't always need to mother and nuture and be wise and call forth the others in my sexy, mystical way." The Amazon represents the great missing link of female energy that has been systematically stripped from our culture for four thousand years and is only now resurging because of economic independence, sexual freedom, and a change in women's awareness of their personal worth.

To be fully alive as a New Age woman, to totally reown our own power, we must be all four types. None of the four aspects must be out of balance. To be totally Amazon would destroy the sensitivity of Eros, the nuturing, loving, mystical qualities that draw forth the heroic powers of the human race. To be only the mother, to be obsessed with the nurturing qualities, means that we would never fully develop our potential and dare to risk taking a stand in the world, developing our independence and internal power. Our struggle as women to attain fitness in health and heart depends on keeping a full balance of the mother, Midean, Hetaera, and Amazon.

It's easy to see why the Amazon quality of women has been so systematically subjugated throughout history. It was Ashley Montague, in writing on the natural superiority of women, who touched on these cultural and social factors:

> Women are just beginning to emerge from their long and unjustified period of subjection. Science has revealed that women are emotionally and constitutionally stronger than men, quicker to respond to stimuli, more resistant to disease, with a lower rate of suicide and alcoholism. Women alone preserve the understanding of love. It's time for them to realize this; time for them to take the world back into their arms so that once again man might know what it means to live within the bosom of the family. Men and women must become partners in the greatest of democratic enterprises, the making of a democratic world.

Many societies were originally matriarchal. Women guided early tribal systems just as the early animal world was guided by the feminine principle. The Amazons were a link between the spirit world and the practical world. As men came to dominate the world in a patriarchal hierarchy, women were subjugated to become the second sex, *subservient to the patriarchal world*. Now the Amazon has to come back. This causes stress in men. They don't understand. But they need to realize that their wholeness as a sex will allow both sexes to be more free. If they are threatened, we can help them understand.

Reowning Your Power

Women need not emulate the male model in sports or in our fitness training. We don't have to compete and dominate in a macho way. We want to create a new model. It must be a model of *spontaneous competance* in which we can at any one moment be mother, Mistrael, Hetaera, Amazon.

As Jeanne said, "In the past, we have become what man wants us to be for his needs. Now women must become what they want to become for their own needs." The voyage of self-growth is painful. If we lean toward to any one of the four female roles, we will get lost. Paul Tillich put it so beautifully: "Joy is the courageous *yes* of the undiscovered part of myself."

The mother, the Midean, and the Mistrael are the women who do not dare be heroines. As little girls, we have limits. We don't go more than two blocks from home. We can't take the bus to get our favorite piece of licorice. Boys don't generally have these limitations to the same extent. When you run, you name your own limits. If you go beyond your limits, it's your responsibility. This is partly related to your sexual freedom as a woman. We don't have to be afraid of impregnation anymore. For the first time in history, we are not limited and it's scary that some women are unwilling to risk the penalities of having no limits. We don't always attain the approval of the men in our lives when we start to assert our independence, no longer merely calling forth their power as the mystical siren.

Daring to be on your own, running for instance, is a symbolic act of awakening the Amazon in you, the whole symbolism of your own power; your own legs carrying you. You're not dependent on anybody else's feet. You're not doing it for anybody else. It's your own locomotion, a marvelous system of your own muscles, body heat, feet. For the rest of your life, you can have your heart break for someone else, take care of someone else, but at this moment you are running for yourself. Whoever heard of Victorian or Medieval women running? Running for women is exploring the unknown. You can't awaken the Amazon by staying in the house and tending to everyone else's needs.

This is a theoretical overview of what you are struggling with as you pass through the revolving doors of your own femininity. Each day you must awaken to redefine who you are and what's important to you. Jung said,

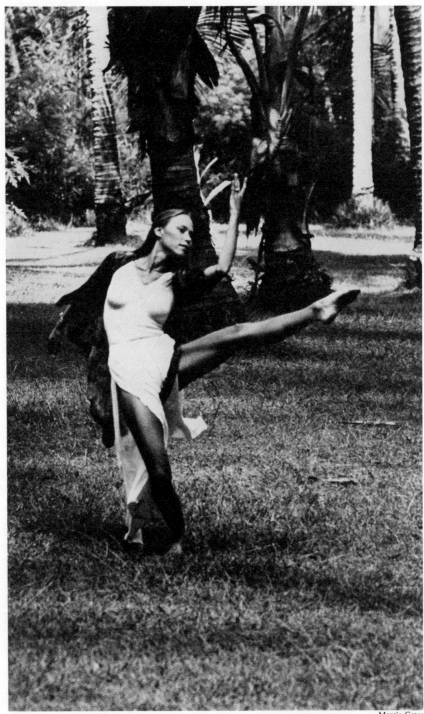

Marcia Cross

"Masculinity in a woman is knowing what you want and going forth to get it." And what I'm trying to share is that knowing what you want and going for it necessitates awakening one aspect of your femininity, the Amazon.

As a small child, I found there was a natural link between the joy of physical movement and the discipline of music. In my own personal journey, I developed an inner sense of my self-worth by playing the edges of my limitations. Life to me was lyrical, rhythmical, and percussive, and as these qualities became interwoven into my life, I began to develop my fourfold femininity. This ultimately led to my career as a New Age Coach.

We all live many lifetimes in one. In the last few years, I've had the privilege of being intimately connected with many women whom I have coached, gotten onto physical training programs, and ultimately brought back from physical and psychological disabilities. I have inspired many to reown their power and to go after a long-dreamed-of career.

Chapter Nine:
Women in Training:
Reowning Your Power

Ernst van Aaken, the great German physician/coach, considered women the true endurance athletes. He clearly articulates the awakening of the *Amazon* spirit as he writes:

> Psychologically, men are more explosive, inconstant, not enduring, and in pain and exertion — especially among high-performance athletes — somewhat sniveling. Women are the opposite: tough, constant, enduring, level and calm under the pain to which their biology exposes them during childbirth. On the average, women are more patient than men. Armed with these advantages, women are in a position to do endurance feats previously considered impossible.

Most of the women I coach are not in touch with a sense of their own endurance when they begin. They generally feel helpless and overly self-critical and tend, at first, to have a real problem maintaining a regular training program. However, once past a trial-and-error period, women generally exhibit incredible tenacity. They are less eager to put undue stress on their bodies and are content to enjoy the training for its own sake, rather than for breaking records or improving distance or time.

Setting up a strong support system is of crucial importance for women in the initial stages of training. In order to have a feeling of progress and success, you should record your experiences in a journal regularly and take time to make a positive appraisal of the changes that are occurring. You can also reach out to others — husbands, lovers, friends, children, neighbors — for support in your training ritual. This sometimes evolves into training groups that meet regularly for dinner or celebration, to encourage one an-

207

other. Be careful, however, not to put so much energy into inspiring the group that you neglect your own training. Make sure you also take time to do training just for yourself. Setting up a regular training ritual complete with rewards is one way of keeping your training going on your own.

When starting a training program, women are sometimes self-conscious about excess weight, sweat, noises, distraction from unknown environmental sources. Worry about others' needs clutters the mind with a stream of chatter. Such mental wandering can be handled by adopting a group spirit. Psychological sharing in a group setting, combined with innerspace work (visualization, imagery, and affirmation), can be used to help express feelings and emotions before and during training. Ending training with a real celebration caps it off. I have found that most resistance, hesitance and fears about body image can be mastered in women's groups. From the beginning, I intuitively structured my groups this way.

For example, in Mill Valley, my women's group met on Thursday nights at 7:00 in a beautiful, inspirational place. There were stained glass windows, thick rugs, soft lights, and a beautiful tiled hot tub and sauna in the back. After our initial sharing session, I would lead the group in innerspace and visualizations. Sometimes we would have flexibility sessions. Then we would go outside and run playfully about the streets of Mill Valley, often doing wind sprints along a straight-away underneath the lights. We would prance up and down the steps of Old Brown's store.

We used props from nature to meditate, such as a plant at the end of a covered wooden walkway. Sometimes we wound up and around the streets in pairs, or did sensing and intuitive training in a grove of redwood trees. Many women brought friends and relatives they wanted to get *hooked*. The group spirit allowed us mutually to support each other's progress and was invaluable in maintaining our training programs.

A Lifestyle Training Program for the women I coach is not merely for putting on or taking off weight. It involves a woman owning her competence and intelligence, assuming her rightful place in society and working to bring about the mass of social changes we need.

One of my close friends, Peggy Taylor, is only 30 years old, but she is the editor of one of the most significant magazines in the country, *New Age Journal*. She is a woman who is owning her competence and intelligence and who wants to do something about the pollutants on our planet. She has found a way to make an impact through the written word. She believes in the importance of affirming oneself.

We met following a story about my work in the *New Age Journal*. Peggy subsequently wanted me to write an article describing my training methods and philosophy. I kept ducking, saying, "Peggy, interview me, you're the writer, you can do it better." She wouldn't accept my opinion and coached me in writing my first article. Peggy *empowered* me to have enough belief in myself to see myself as a "writer." In turn, we had several running sessions around a beautiful reservoir and park in Newton, Massachusetts, and I introduced her to the joys of running. Peggy and I have talked at length about women reowning their power as part of the New Age consciousness. Peggy said:

> We are in transition on this planet. The human race can destroy itself very easily. We are at that point in history where we must either evolve to some other level or destroy a large part of civilization. The institutions that are perpetuating nuclear power, those that are ripping people off, are losing a lot of their power. There is a growing grassroots movement that is getting stronger every year. At the magazine, we are trying to show that what *you* do, makes a difference. And, if you choose to do nothing, *that* makes a difference. We're trying to empower people.
>
> As a woman I was afraid to share my feelings, especially negative, because of fear of being rejected. I've learned to articulate my feelings with non-authoritarian expression without unconsciously falling into patterns of submission. *Personal truthfulness has a real power.* I find that when I tell the truth as I see it, it opens a door. I have learned to share without dumping and so I don't end up hurting people. This gives me a sense of my own strength. The keys to managing stress are the ability to look at how you perpetuate a situation, and learning to express our feelings openly and truthfully.
>
> When I assert myself, I can feel my spine straighten. "I *won't* have the planet polluted." And I *won't* have someone treat me with a degrading attitude.

The social concerns I'm most interested in are the role of sports, games, and physical education in shaping our consciousness toward our planet and our bodies. Women have an opportunity to redefine sports and games in our culture, to assume their rightful place in inspiring participation and minimizing competition. This idea is receiving more support from experts in the field, all too familiar with the destructive effects of competition.

Dr. Thomas Tutko, the coordinator of the Institute for the Study of Athletic Motivation in San Jose, California, believes that women can and should start over and create more effective role models in sports than the "winners" model, which has come from the male model based upon competition.

"Women are at the crossroads of sports history," he says. "They can develop a new, healthy, vigorous and psychologically stable model based on participation instead of winning at all costs. Or they can go into competitive athletics as men have done, which is saying in essence that the male model is right. "And that," Dr. Tutko maintains, "would be stupid." ("Play to Win", by Jane Leavy, *Harper's*.)

Taking Charge of Your Body

The first step in reowning your power is to take charge of your body. Your ultimate goal is to find work that challenges and inspires, work that makes your feel creative and inventive; a full participant in this wondrous new age of rebirth and reawakening on our planet. Women must persist as leaders and teach the way of harmony, balance, and love.

But you will never surface in the world and help bring about this different kind of energy unless you're internally powerful. And developing this internal power can only happen when you have a vital reserve of physical and spiritual energy to draw on. It takes sheer endurance and discipline to carry on the multiplicity of functions and roles that are demanded of us during this incredible period of transition.

It's pretty easy to spot a woman who is on a physical training program. She moves with a bounce. Her eyes are clear. There's a sleek leanness about her. It is easier for her to get things done. A woman who is running two to three miles a day and doing yoga several times a week finds it easier to cope with a strenuous job and still take care of the myriad demands that fall on women.

But women often find it hard to articulate the psychological freedom that accompanies the reowning of their physical power. In this chapter, I am going to show you, through several case studies, what it means to physically train your body. You will see the emotional changes that result when you train your body, not with the goal of being a sex object so as to be better able to manipulate the world, but with the goal of having the energy to take on your share of planetary responsibility.

Psychological freedom makes it possible for you to do what you want to do in the way you want to do it. When you have psychological freedom, you make decisions and execute those decisions with a positive attitude and force. You are confident that you can master the unknowns and fulfill your expectations, rather than fitting your energies to suit everybody else's needs and expectations.

The real significance of psychological therapies is the way they help people unhook themselves from *playing the victim*: "I can't do this because of that." The basis of Gestalt therapy is *taking responsibility*. Once a woman truly understands that she can decide what she wants to do with her life and that she can execute her desires in a way that will give her joy, pleasure, and satisfaction, she will start to become a transformed human being.

The key tool in reowning your power is the training of your will; training your intentionality systematically and using it skillfully and wisely, and extending it to include a sense of oneness with the life force of the universe.

A daily running program, a flexibility program, and proper nutrition are the next steps. As you prepare yourself physically and psychologically, you will see that having a meaningful job need not be just an idle dream. You will be prepared to pursue your wildest dream.

Beginning a Woman's Fitness Program

If you have never been on a systematic training program before, you should take the following steps.

First, get a hair sample analysis and find out about your biochemistry. (See Chapter 6.) You need first and foremost to clean up your nutrition and make sure that you're not getting foods into your diet that will destroy all your motivation and energy. You need foods that will help you sustain an increasing stress load from your physical endurance training.

Second, get the book *The Light Of Yoga* by Alice Christensen and David Rankin (See the References) and begin to do the flexibility exercises explained in it. The book is a marvelous introduction to exercises you can do in your home. These exercises can help you get more oxygen to your cells as well as help you begin training your will. Early some morning, find the most beautiful place in your house, put on some music, and go through Christianson's book. It will take you about 30 minutes.

Third, begin either walking or running or a combination for 20 minutes, three times a week. Get a friend to go with you at least once a week. Gradually extend this to four or five times a week at 30 to 40 minutes per time. It will be necessary for you to buy a proper pair of shoes. You should always run in the most inspiring environment in your neighborhood.

Fourth, use a tape recorder to make training tapes. Get the book *The Act of Will* by Roberto Assagiolli. Familiarize yourself with its theoretical base.

Fifth, purchase some inexpensive equipment that can be used in your home. Get a jumprope, a small trampoline (a good indoor model costs about $125), a slant board, and a strength building device such as the Stretch-ur (which sells for about $13). You might move into a set of small weights, but only when your body is aligned.

Sixth, read three books on nutrition: Pavao Airola's *Are You Confused?*, Leonard and Pritikin's, *Live Longer Now*, and Francis Lappee's, *Diet for a Small Planet*. Start to get salt, oils, fats, sugars, coffee, tea, alcohol out of your diet. And of course, eliminate cigarettes and dope. Don't cook food in aluminum pans: aluminum is a metal which can cause premature aging and is toxic to our bodies. Use *stainless steel* or cast iron cooking utensils exclusively, as Teflon and ceramic chips go into the food.

Seventh, study the chapter on Innerspace and start to do some of the visualizations and concentration exercises.

Seven Key Training Procedures for Women

In my training approach, men and women basically do the same things, but with a difference on emphasis. Here I want to highlight seven key procedures to which women need to give special attention.

First, and most important, is to make your daily training program top priority. You must make everything and everybody else bend to that program. Even if you only have 20 minutes twice a week to begin with, that's fine. It's a start. But whatever the time is, it must be put ahead of everything else. Women are involved in so many humanistic and caring activities that this becomes hard. Women feel such responsibility for others, they neglect their obligations to themselves. Taking time out for a daily training program may make them feel guilty when there is laundry to be folded, a boss to report to, a child to be fed, a committee meeting to attend. *Your time for running, swimming, stretching, or meditating must be seen as vitally important, just as important as feeding a child or getting someone to a doctor.*

You must decide that for six weeks, training will be your priority. You will never have to look far for reasons why you can't train today. It's true that clothes need to be ironed, appointments need to be kept, business deals need to be closed. But how can we build a different society, how can we connect to our life force, if we don't prepare ourselves with the daily ritual of training? This means cardiovascular, flexibility, strength, and inner-space work. For just six weeks, put training first. The difference you feel will convince you that new energy will be released and all those other things will still get done.

Second, keep a personal assessment profile. Constantly project the image of what you want for yourself and *don't be afraid to go after it.*

Third, fill your environment with energizing statements of love, hope, joy, beauty and wisdom. Put colorful, inspiring posters and sayings on your walls. And for each statement that you put on the wall by somebody else, put up a statement that you have written yourself. Make a training tape for yourself. Write down affirmations concerning what you desire for yourself. "I (give your name) strongly desire (state your desire)." Then turn on your tape recorder and record them. Express on that tape exactly how you want to see your life in six months, one year, three years, five years.

Fourth, create a support group. Surround yourself with friends, especially women, who have *positive vibrations* and who will reflect back to you your uniqueness. Because our culture is basically oriented toward competition, not art, we have had little or no experience using sports and games to awaken the feminine aspects of our psyche. Having your own small training group could make the difference in whether or not your training program succeeds.

Fifth, stop worrying about whether you're as attractive as you might be. Bring that energy inside and focus on going about your day *as if* you already are that which you desire. Project it, believe it, and discipline it.

Sixth, if you're afraid of letting go of some relationship that you are hanging on to, take a good look at your fear. Start to imagine what it would be like to support yourself emotionally and financially in a positive and reinforcing atmosphere.

Seventh, Make a serious beginning on cleaning up your nutrition.

Mary and the Marathon

Mary Owen is a 37-year-old woman who like Peggy underwent major lifestyle changes. Following a workshop, we had dinner together and she decided that she was going to become Mary, athlete in training, and train for the Boston Marathon. She had been really athletic as a young girl. After she married she stayed home for ten years to support her husband in furthering his professional advancement. Finally, she decided to go out on her own. Her former husband now has custody of their children and she has just remarried.

A couple of years ago I went through a really deep change inside when I became aware that I was not at the helm of my own life. I realized that even though I was trying very hard and doing all the things that I thought were right, part of me didn't feel as if I had control over my own life. At the time I was a single parent with two kids, trying to have a relationship and work at the same time.

I was running here and there. I went through a lot of quiet time; a lot of time sitting and thinking. I started running. I've run on and off for about six years, though never consistently. I find that just getting out there and running is something that clears my head. One day I ran by a store and saw a poster about a workshop you were giving. It said that running is related to total life and can transform your total experience. It seemed to fit right in with what I was feeling.

I had been straining in my running. The workshop was to help make it fun. I wanted to see if that was possible. I wanted to find bouncier, looser ways to help me enjoy running. The workshop opened new doors for me. When I saw you next November, I was running about five miles a day and had run one race, the Bonne Bell. I felt very excited about it.

In the back of my mind, I wondered if I could ever run the marathon. I remember saying to you one evening at dinner, "Coach, I'm running five miles a day. Do you think by next April I'll be ready to run 26?" You said, "Sure." I made a real commitment to do it. I took your advice about making a chart on the wall. I put the time I woke up, what the day was like, what I ate, what exercises I did, how far I ran, how long I ran, and/or if I played squash. I put down what my mood was and how I felt physically and emotionally. I would keep the chart very meticulously, but there would be days when I would feel so low that I didn't want to record anything about my life. But on the whole I kept enough so that I could see what my life was like from November to February.

During my training, I'd wake up in the morning and not want to get out of bed. It was a challenge for me to try to run earlier and earlier in the morning because at that time the air was a lot cleaner. But then there was another part of me that wanted to snuggle and stay in bed. I had to work out running and being with someone. It was a matter of balancing. Lou was always supportive but it was hard for me socially to feel that I could just take my own life and do whatever I wanted to do, no matter who else was around. Yet not having the children for the first time, I could explore more of the possibility of getting out.

But of course, that's what the whole thing is about; learning how to be yourself with someone else. I still feel that it is a challenge to learn how to integrate all I want to do in life with another person. It was an internal challenge this whole winter to keep my purpose clear. It was nice to see how, when I didn't live up to my training standards or when I ate bad food, I wouldn't judge myself negatively. I could see myself not accomplishing my purpose and just see it as a fact. I would just say that approach doesn't feel right to me, instead of being negative about it. And then I would get back on the track.

Each day I would run between eight and nine miles. I ran about an hour and 25 to 45 minutes. Some days I'd run two hours and then the next day an hour and 20 minutes. I tried to make an internal pacing. About one day out of seven or eight I wouldn't run. And sometimes not for two or three days. But it felt so good to get back into running and felt so awful when I didn't run. It became a kind of addiction. The dawn was just coming up when I ran. It wasn't ever dangerous. I found all the back roads in Brookline.

On the day of the marathon Lou, my second husband, and Tony, my son, took me out to Hopkinton. It was very exciting to see all the people around. Everybody was doing their warm-ups. I was so excited to be in that lineup. I was way at the back because I hadn't officially qualified. There was jovial laughter and excitement all around. Starting off, we walked for five minutes because there were so many people. So it was after the starting line that our group began breaking into a long slow jog. It was a perfect start.

There was elation among everybody running. The people along the side were so supportive. They'd hand out oranges and water and give encouragement. I made contact with people's eyes and got spurts of energy from them. I knew my friends would be waiting near the end. As I got closer to Boston they started to appear and run along with me. Some of them joined me at the beginning of Heartbreak Hill and ran up the hill with me. I didn't even realize it was Heartbreak Hill, I was so excited.

There were times around the eight or nine mile mark that my legs were really stiff. Then at the halfway point I realized if I wanted to walk or exercise I could do that. I didn't have any rules. But I began to think that maybe I could run this thing without ever walking. Just before Heartbreak Hill I realized I was feeling very stiff. I loosened up my running and thought of energy flowing through me. I didn't resist the pain, I just went with it. And it went away. In the last half, I would go in and out of experiencing pain, but I knew I was going to make it. So I just experienced how it felt.

The most exciting moment was near the end. The crowd was way back and there was a wide track to the finish line. We went around the last few corners and people were cheering wildly. The last person participating in the wheelchair marathon was going through the finish line. There was a big cheer for him. And then I went through and there was Lou waiting with open arms.

Running has been very important to me. The part of myself that has needed the most integration is accepting my own power. People told me for a long time that they perceive me as being powerful. But it's a whole other thing to experience myself in that way in a clear, purposeful manner. Running has given me a chance to experience and explore all that I could do. Power and discipline were both qualities that I really wanted to know were mine.

Mary went about her training in a sensible way. First, she came to a workshop and got the theoretical and practical background she needed from a woman she thought she could trust. She learned how to monitor her body and adopted a playful attitude. She embarked on a program of self-knowledge and nutrition. She reowned her power on a base of psychological freedom and developed her masculine energies without relinquishing her feminine energies.

The Yin and the Yang

There are two basic principles governing the universe, the Yin and the Yang, the logos and the eros. We all have a receptive, nurturing, yin aspect to our natures and a physical, powerful, hunter's yang aspect as well. Jung called these the female, or eros, aspect, and the male, or logos, aspect. Each of us has both female and male hormones in our chemistries. Each of us likes to dominate at times, just as each of us likes to relinquish at times. Trouble starts in a person of either sex when one side subsumes the other. To be healthy, we must integrate these two sides.

Characteristically the male has been more logos in his mode of functioning, more thinking, more discriminating. Logos comes from *agitar*, meaning *to agitate*. When we think, we agitate things together. Logos concentrates on seeing the facts, sorting out, discriminating and eliminating the unnecessary.

The eros principle deals with relatedness and is characteristically a more female function. Women are usually more comfortable relating to people, bringing people and parts together. But they often have a difficult time discriminating. Jung believed that these basic distinctions were culturally, not biologically, determined. Because our culture had to produce, it became achievement oriented. The logos principle has reigned for thousands of years. The male who could not hone, refine, sort out, could not compete well. It's very easy to see why men with their superior physical abilities soon dominated the universe.

The eros principle has been culturally subjugated to the more dominant male-oriented logos. The far side of any quality is neurosis and we have a neurotically tipped logos culture based on money, power, competition. Very little of our culture is guided by loving relatedness. True creativity, comfort, self-actualization, come when a woman or man is able to blend these two modes of functioning and swing between the polarities.

Health for a women, then, is first and foremost being able to develop abilities and talents highly enough to function in both realms. That is what androgyny is. The sexes have been caught between two polarities. The far side of either is illness. Logos for women means knowing what you want and going forth to get it; being clear, sorting out, eliminating garbage, taking a stand. But we must balance this with eros, our relatedness, our sensitivity, honoring intuition and being nuturing, but not being caught in a "swamp of relatedness."

As Jeanne Gibbs said, "When I go to my lake, I relinquish both my eros and my logos. I have no achievement, no relatedness needs. The inner wholeness springs forth, a blend of the Yin and the Yang, the eros and the logos. It happens freely. I get in touch with the spirit world, the stumps, the water, the mountains. All have a life unto themselves. It's their world and they permit me to enter it. All the elements have a spirit. It's a mystical and symbolic world. I feel connected to the infinity of life."

I believe that our woman's gift of eros, love relatedness energy, leads us more naturally into the spiritual aspect of life. It is usually men who have written about these concepts throughout history, because of their ability to articulate ideas logically and succinctly. Women have been closer to the spirit world, the essential wisdom of the universe, the intuitive sense of life. We have a greater responsibility now to develop not only the four aspects of femininity but also to balance our Yin and Yang, our logos and eros.

When I coach women I draw out the balance of their androgynous nature by awakening their inner physical power and helping them overcome tendencies of too much nesting and passivity, or blindly following the leadership of a man.

A New Age Executive

Rose Thorne, like Mary, saw the importance of taking charge of her body. Rose is the 30-year-old codirector of Interface, a nonprofit educational association in Boston which sponsors workshops, lectures, and conferences on health and education. She has evolved into a New Age woman and in the process has taken along her profession, her marriage, her physical training, her spiritual awareness, and her vision of a better world. She went from a position of *maintaining* to one of *initiating*. In the process, she experienced a whole metamorphosis. She is a New Age woman executive who is also an athlete in training.

> At the time I became codirector, Interface was not well organized nor financially stable. My energy had been dissipated by the chaos of the operation and it was difficult working with the men. But now that's changed. I'm working with another woman and it's wonderful. We have a very different approach to the work. For the first time, I feel in control. Until this point I was completely frustrated because I was powerless.

Though I was completely committed to my work and feeling tremendous responsibility for it, I had no authority to change the situation and felt swept along in a tumultuous operation.

There's a real sense of freedom to be in power and in control. However, it's also very awesome and frightening because you have the weight of the organization completely on you. In the past, I could feel that if the organization didn't work, the consequences would fall on somebody else. Now, it's somewhat frightening and tension-producing to have that constant feeling that I'm in control and responsible for the whole operation. And there are time I feel that I just can't do it. I get tongue-tied, scared. I feel completely overwhelmed.

Right now, I am so aware that my being is much more than my body. There's such a sense of my divine connection and divine purpose in this lifetime, and I feel compelled to do good work and provide these services for others. I also have a sense of being a perishable vessel of energy attempting to get through this difficult classroom that we call life and do it well. That's what gets me through. I meditate on my connection with the universe and try to open up to my higher self and get inner guidance.

My running is a form of meditation and a time when I commune with nature and feel enveloped with divine energy, peace, and love. I try to take that energy with me to my work.

While I'm involved in other sports, running is my love. I sometimes think it would be better not to be so singular, but it's hard for me to do anything but run. I find it is the most intoxicating, attractive endeavor that I've ever come across. I've been running for about five years. I had stopped smoking and was nervous and highly strung. I realized that I was feeling terrible. I was having skin problems which I never had in my whole life. I couldn't figure out what was wrong.

Then I realized that I had always run when I was younger. I had been very involved in athletics and did a lot of sweating. But I had lost sight of the benefit of physical exercise. One day I just bolted out of the house and began to sprint. At that time, running wasn't the fad it is now. There were very few women runners. I ran with a woman friend and the abuse that we used to suffer was just unmentionable. I had spent five years feeling terrible all the time. But as soon as I started running, my life literally changed.

When I took your workshop, whole new dimensions were opened for me. Other interests of mine such as spiritual awareness, meditation, and a sense of communicating with my environment were integrated into running. When you introduced me to those things as well as the endurance aspect of training, it completely changed my life. Before I would just run. I did no stretching. Now I always do yoga in the morning or at night. Running has changed my level of energy. I went from being listless and exhausted to being absolutely full of energy all day long.

I do about four miles a day. If I don't run one day, I'll do four miles the next day. Ideally, I run early in the morning. The air is clean. The environment is not polluted with noise. I run on the Esplanade along the Charles River. If I run after work, I go to Fresh Pond. Neither place is ideal because they're both next to highways. But there are trees, so I figure it's better than some other places.

There's definitely a connection between my running and my new-found power as an executive. The sense of strength and endurance that I've gotten out of my running has naturally spilled over into my work. Running gives me a tremendous sense of my physical strength. It really contributes to my capactity to take on more and more responsibilities. I have to say that my running gives me a sense of total regeneration. It's meditative and gives me the peace and strength to do my work. When I don't run, I can feel my energy go into an immediate decline.

And I really do relish the fact that I am so strong. My husband is not used to being with a woman who is as physically strong as I am. The people I work with regard it as pretty unusual. For women who want to succeed as executives, I'd strongly recommend some kind of physical endeavor that will develop a sense of purpose and discipline. And with purpose and discipline you can do anything you want.

Women must learn that they are safe. I know I'm constantly overwhelmed with fear and a sense of inadequacy. I try to transcend that kind of perception and energy. Getting into a physical endeavor gives people a sense of themselves, a sense of their completeness as people, a sense that they are safe. As a woman I have constantly felt insecure. But at long last I'm starting to feel some sense of relief from that emotion.

I felt insecure because I was dependent on other people for a sense of myself. I never had a sense of authority in a situation. I've always had the responsibility but never the authority. Also, our cultural education as women causes us to seek our identity through things external to ourselves, e.g., men.

Rose is an extremely emotional and sensual person, but at the same time has great organizational ability and efficiency while retaining a tender, feminine side. It is important that we as women don't lose this. Rose says,

You put me in touch with that. Interface put me in touch with that. What it amounts to is *nurturing*. And women shouldn't shy away from that. It's a very powerful notion. Interface had been in its death throes because no one was nurturing it. No one had the concept of it being something above and beyond us. It was like this infantile being that needed to be nurtured. Everyone was thinking of how it was going to serve them and promote them. What we do now is nurture it as women. It is curious because we are nurturing it and, coincidentally, we are women.

Physically appreciating your body, loosing weight, and having a daily training ritual with emphasis on training your will to open transpersonal values are inextricably woven with enjoying your sexuality and manifesting your dormant capacities and talents to the world. Your increasing sense of the unity of all mankind with all living things, i.e., cosmic consciousness, your feelings of mastery and relinquishing patterns, masochism, and weakness are all as important to you psychologically as physical training is to your health and vitality. You are not only training your body, you are training your consciousness to believe in yourself.

Women I Have Coached

What kind of women come to me for training? Here are some typical examples.

Marcia, a diabetic, had a consultation with Chuck Richardson, a physicist and exercise physiologist, and me. We talked about the effects of insulin injections on her physiological system and about going on a vegetarian diet. After several coaching sessions, she began to extricate herself from a destructive love relationship and to overcome negative eating habits. She is now working as a television producer.

Pattie was hooked into lifestyle of pathological narcissism which had consumed from $40,000 to $60,000 in therapist fees. With the help of a Lifestyle Training Program, she has begun to come out of a childlike relationship with her husband and is now teaching classes and opening her own business.

Anne, a 40-year-old nurse, following an emotional explosion at a retreat I conducted at Westerbeck Ranch, quit her job in a surgical operating room. She could no longer bear to see some doctors with polluted, toxified bodies carving up people and dumping poisonous chemicals down the waste system. She is now a student and teacher of holistic medicine.

Andrea, a 30-year-old mother, had undergone shots and surgery for severe depressions and feelings of helplessness. Through a Lifestyle Assessment and Hair Sample Analysis it was determined that she was pre-diabetic. She has begun to overcome this by proper nutrition, meditation, and physical training.

Pat Ellsberg is a radiant, socially aware woman whom I have coached in tennis and running. She used my classes to test her teaching abilities. With Pat laying the base, I was able to get her husband, Daniel, on a training program. He now runs six miles a day.

From Cosmic Wisdom to Internal Trust

Biological Cycles

One of the reasons for the volcanic eruption in the psyches of women today is that at the deepest biochemical level they are relinquishing their previous modes of survival: assuming the mother role, being protected by the man, being in a subservient position owing to economic dependency. The cataclysmic changes women are experiencing require a balancing of the feminine *nurturing* energies with the masculine *take-charge* energies needed for survival in the business and political worlds.

Women are prepared to balance these energies because their entire bio-chemistry is governed by the cycles of the moon; the menstrual cycle that links them to Universal Law in a way which a man very rarely experiences. Her emotional states are influenced by the water balances in her body just as the tides of the ocean are drawn by the cycles of the moon.

There is something very dramatic about a flow of blood coming from a woman's body. We can watch a seed grow into a life. This experience provides a linkage between women and the universe. And the universality of this connection can have a profound political effect in restructuring the consciousness of the New Age.

It is absolutely imperative for a woman to stay in touch with and reinforce her biological link to the cosmos. I feel that I haven't succeeded in my work with a woman until I've fully awakened that feeling of universal connection with all womanhood. This will be one of the foundation stones of the New Age.

Overcoming Self-Consciousness

In your training, some of your experiences will be less than cosmic. I recall once running exhaustedly through a damp San Francisco park before day-break and suddenly screaming as I planted my flying foot on the belly of a snoring drunk. It was probably just as frightening for him as for me, for I am no dainty dolly. His woodland respite was interrupted by 145 muscular pounds of blonde Valkyrie leaping on his stomach.

Another time, Mike Spino and I were chased by a drunk with a broken bottle when we were running along the Embarcadero waterfront early one morning. He turned and ran for us, thinking we were chasing him and I almost ran smack into a forklift truck. The amused driver yelled "I'll get him."

I have often stopped traffic when stretching a sore ligament. I've been whistled at when I stopped to tie a leotard because I was sweating so hard it had come loose. I've been honked at, yelled at to "keep it up, lady." I've been chased by motorboats while swimming, even had harpoon boats come out after me when sharks were around. I've been startled by an unknown intruder while shouting out my ideals during a run, bitten by dogs, and chased by property owners. I once collapsed exhausted at a coffee shop and had to borrow 25 cents for a cup of tea. I've even hitch-hiked home when I've injured myself or got lost or have gone out too far.

A strong sense of humor is especially important at the beginning of training. You will be self-conscious about the subcutaneous layer of fat that distresses you so much. Oddly, that fat can be your secret source of power. Women in marathon races often start slowly and eventually surpass men in contests reminiscent of the old fable of the tortoise and the hare.

An article in *Medical World News*, August 25, 1975, reviewed findings of Dr. Joan Ullyot, an M.D. and an accomplished marathoner. Although male track stars are notoriously skinny, Ullyot says, this is not so with women.

For example, Eileen Waters, record holder of the 50 mile race for women, flucturates between 135 and 150 pounds at 5 feet 3 inches. Waters starts slowly and speeds up as much as 25 per cent by the end of the race.

According to the article, Dr. Ullyot suspects that "All other things being equal, a women of the same size and age as a man weighs less because fat is lighter than muscle mass and she can go farther because fat is a better fuel and she has more of it."

Overcoming Youthful Indulgences

I believe it was George Bernard Shaw who once said, "It's too bad youth is wasted on the young." How many of us look back on our overindulgences and follies with deep regret, saying, "If I had only known better." Sometimes youth gains wisdom early thus avoiding an unfulfilled lifetime. A lovely 21-year-old, speaking of the physical abuse of her body, said:

> For several years, I didn't care. I smoked two packs of Camel cigarettes a day, drank lots of coffee, lots of alcohol. I tried to subdue the natural power of my body because I was afraid of it. In some ways I was dying. I was not in control of my will. I was at the end of my youth and I decided that I was killing the most vital, vivacious, spirited flame of my being because I was afraid of its power to succeed."

I was looking at the slim, beautiful body, the silken hair, the green cat eyes set off by a Hawaiian suntan. I was sitting across the couch from my own daughter, Terry.

I asked how she saw physical discipline in terms of taking responsibility for her power. I also asked how her current mode of natural, healthful living had evolved from her inner needs and what part her love of music and dance played in this transition. I wanted to know what the turning point was.

> I began to realize that the body truly is the temple of the spirit. This body that I carry with me is in essence my daily lesson to heighten my spiritual goal, and eventually I won't need this body. It will have completed its purpose. The body to me is a complete teacher. It has its own language, its own way of operating through life. It has its own control systems. I personally don't know how it survives and yet it does. Day in and day out it serves me. So the least I can do is serve it. The least I can do is care for my life force. If not, why am I here? I value my evolution on this planet more than I value individual gain. So my body is the extension of my spirit. It is the outer shell of my inner being and it shines when I shine.

> I feel I have a mission in life now to be the fullest human being I can. To be a woman in the New Age means to have control of the choices I can make and not feel victimized by my emotions. It's my own path and no one can start it for me. I value honesty. My deepest dreams and desires

have changed. I want to perfect my art of movement and dance as a form of self-healing. Freedom to me means an inner state of true knowledge. Knowledge is freedom. I wasn't free before. I was a victim of my own indulgences. But I had to accept and love myself where I was, not feel I had wasted my life. Now I too want to ignite others to own their inner power through dance and natural living because I know what's it's like not to be there.

I must admit, as a mother, I feel honored that my daughter has joined a path similar to mine completely from a self-directed place. We often work as a team in conducting workshops and clinics. We do multi-media artistic events together in which she dances and I improvise music interspersed with physical training and the teaching of natural health practices.

Taking Responsibility

Most women have a tendency to try to latch on to experts. There is a political and social causation involved. We have centuries of infantile dependency imbedded in our legal system and social norms. There is much for a woman to overcome. And I urge women to start to look to themselves for answers dealing with their health and vitality.

From the very beginning, I try to turn the responsibility for training over to the woman herself as much as possible. I try to mirror back her lifestyle in such a way that the full responsibility for conceiving, designing, implementing, and maintaining the training program comes from within her own psyche. I hardly know a woman I've coached who has not made marked changes in her life at this point as a direct result of "reowning her power."

Many women are used to authority figures telling them what to do, when to do it, how to do it. They feel that they have little control of things. My approach is to put responsibility in their laps in such a way that they are not overwhelmed. They need to know that they can take things into their own hands and make changes themselves. And this is where training the will is of such importance. It's one thing for them to understand and desire to take control, and another thing to maintain that control.

Vinita Reowns Her Power

My chief woman assistant, Vinita, is a 35-year-old physical education teacher. A few years ago, she came to a Tennis Flow Workshop I was teaching for the University of California Berkley Extension Center. She was shy, yet her tennis game revealed a personal radiance and expressiveness. Within two days I *knew* she was to be my long-awaited assistant.

Once, during that workshop, I bombarded her with balls from the net while another person hit balls to her from the baseline. She was to return everything she could get to. Sweat streaming down, she bounded with lightning reflexes and accelerated her response pattern as demanded by the exercise. She practiced meditation in between, to be centered and to increase instant kinesthetic response to the pace of too many balls. When she returned to regular play, her *internal time sense* remained and there was a marked improvement in her tennis game. The technique of acceleration of tempo interspersed with meditation, *seed thoughts* (e.g., "I am centered and graceful.") and visualizations had a remarkable effect. For Vinita this was the beginning of "reowning her power."

In the past two years, I have watched her psyche open up, revealing hidden talents and gifts. Once, after a mountain run, she meditated on "the message that came to her from the spirit of an animal." I have watched her take innovative methods of training to her students in high school. I have seen her inner power grow as she follows a daily training program. And she now teaches some of my university courses.

This once-shy, rather self-doubting woman is emerging as a leader and spokeswoman, becoming a new breed of coach, holistic health educator, and spiritual voyager. She is now teaching in the Physical Arts program at Meadowlark and is a New Age Coach.

Women with Children

Donna, A Young Mother in the East

Donna, a 30-year-old mother, started a training program after being inspired by watching all the women runners out in the streets during a bitter winter. During this time she was helping me type and correct the manuscript for this book and she became more interested in training. As Donna explained:

> I felt the need for a training program because I wasn't as physically active as I should be. My weight has been redistributed after having children. My stomach muscles and thighs were soft. But the trend this year has been to running. It's becoming a new way of life for people. Just watching people run by your house makes you feel that *if she can do it, so can I*. Maybe I'll feel better. I've wondered if I was lazy or neglectful. I finally asked, "Why not be in the best possible physical shape you can?" I realized that I could get into a pattern and incorporate the children. If they could come with me shopping, they could come with me for a physical workout. It's just a matter of adapting yourself to something new in your schedule.
>
> I have one friend with four children, and she does ice skating, coasting and walking with them. She packs them up with hats, mittens, boots, snowsuits, scarves, and takes them out. We did that this winter with our sled. We really made use of it with all the snow in January and February. Several times we did our grocery shopping with the sled. We had a one-

> week ban on driving cars after a blizzard and we learned to do without them. It was very nice and peaceful. Arlington looked like an Alpine village. There were people going to the post office on skis. There were men pulling little children on sleds and mothers pulling groceries on sleds. One day we walked over a telphone booth, that's how high the snow was.

She continued by equating her feelings towards running with aesthetics:

> There is a feeling of freedom when you run through a grass field or a park; almost like running away from your cares, the yelling and screaming of children in the backyard. It is just getting off on your own. It is similar to painting. Sometimes when I'm painting, I feel as if I'm in a different world. I get so involved that I lose track of time and at the end I feel I've accomplished something. There's almost a spiritual awakening in running. Getting in good physical health must cleanse your mind. Mothers listening to little children all day need to have time alone to *think*. We need to support each other. We could take turns caring for each other's children.

Donna's training goals are ambitious. She wants to ride her bike at least an hour per day, exercise at home at least half an hour, and run an hour also. She has her family on a good nutritional program and casually mentioned that her children now reach for an apple, orange, pear, or raw vegetable rather than sweets and candy. "Many times my daughter will give a lollipop back to me after a lick or two. Sometimes I think her body is rejecting sweets."

An increasing number of young mothers are, like Donna, becoming *aware*. They are setting an example for their family and building a lifestyle around physical exercise, despite cold winters, the hassle of bundling up children to get them outside and making arrangements with friends. They are leaping quite a few hurdles to become *athletes in training*.

Carolyn, A Young Mother in California

Carolyn is a good example of how women can affect the consciousness of the New Age. In this case, it is a family. Imagine what can happen when this energy spreads to the larger family of humanity.

> When Carolyn first came to me, she was worried about her weight. She had tried everything from diets to shots to sporadic physical training. As a mother, she was worried about finding care for her young son while she trained. I suggested that she take him along to the field. Although Carolyn still treasures the frequent times she is able to run alone, she and her young son have had wonderful hours of sharing together. "He claps his hands and runs in place while I soar past him on the dirt track. Now when he sees me put on my training clothes, he begs to go along."

> I fondly remember the day her husband, Charles, cheered her on from the bleachers, holding their son and beaming with pride in Carolyn's newfound physical pursuit. As she and I swept around the track, Carolyn

announced that she was entering her first race. "Even if I come in last, it won't matter."

Later, Charles told me, "It's really a reversal now. Several mornings a week, while I'm still in bed, Carolyn gets up to train. I was always the *big athlete*, now it's Carolyn. Actually, *she's* inspired me. I just have to get this knee of mine fixed. I was running in my heavy army boots. She got me out of them and into some good, light running shoes. She got me off the pavement and onto the grass. Here I am, a PhD psychologist, and doing the damnedest, most stupid thing; training the way I did in the army and damaging my body. Carolyn is becoming *my coach*."

Women in Motion

Helen, A Mentalist, Discovers the Body

One of my busiest clients is the well-known Berkeley psychic, Helen Palmer. Helen had no interest in her body. Primarily a mentalist, she viewed the body as an unwelcome encumbrance that interfered with her mystical and spiritual world. But now Helen trains an hour a day. Why? Because it improves her capacity for work. Helen says:

Since I started to train, there's less of me than there used to be and I feel a lot better. But the major effect is on my work. I used to crash in the evening. I would resort to hypnosis if I had an evening appointment in order to raise my energy. Now I can do it without hypnosis by using physical activity as a way of generating energy.

Helen was so reclusive, so private, so devoted to her family and her work that she rarely ventured outside her house. Because she goes into low-energy, low-metabolism states during the readings that she gives most of the day, she needed physical activity to balance her sedentary life. When she asked me to help her devise a personal training program, our challenge was to find a routine Helen could do within her house. She was so averse to going outside that we had to set up a specific time of day for her to walk down the front steps of her house and up and down the street in front of it.

The rest of her training program was composed of exercising, running up and down stairs, and jumping rope, all at home. Helen is not fond of exercise for its own sake. She gets her pay-off in the improvement of her general level of health and her ability to do more work. She now grudgingly admits she is enjoying it more than she used to. When I told Helen several months ago that I had a dream about her running up and down the hills of Berkeley, the very thought was absurd to her. She laughed. Now she climbs the hill in back of her house to go for an hour's daily work-out at a local public gymnasium. She has even made the step of moving from the house in which she lived for many years. Her wan cheeks have a slight flush, her rounded arms are firmer, and the quiet good humor I saw in her before has become a charming drollery. Helen analyzes herself:

I'm a mentalist, so I sort of put down the body. When it gets tired, or I really get sick, my reaction is one of disgust at myself. I don't like illness in myself or in other people. In my earlier life, I was an intellectual. It seemed to me that the great people, the ones that really had it together, the great minds, were the ones who had it together intellectually. Most of the people I admired were totally disinterested in their bodies. I realize now that this idea is not true, but only a matter of my own projection.

When I was much younger, I was a dancer, and I thought the body was the crowning glory. But I found that I was a mentalist and my tendency is to evaluate a single thing as the best. I could forget about the body because I had moved into the intellect. I could very easily discredit intellectualism now because I've moved into intuition. That has to do with me, not the way it is. I would like to get rid of my body, get rid of intellectualism, and just go into the intuitive space. But of course you can't do that without a vehicle.

I have an intuition that I cannot afford to just be intuitive all day long. My physical system will simply deteriorate sooner than it should. I look ten years younger now than when I started training a few months ago. For me, the weak link in my energy system is the body. If I don't exercise my body, I could get old before my time and be an extremely obese and cold psychic, shivering my way to enlightenment. I don't think you can make the jump into a real enlightening experience unless you have tremendous stamina.

The reason that training was intially agonizing for me was that it hit me in all the wrong spaces. It's exposure. As soon as I started to run, I instantly thought everyone was looking at me, when actually, people were just running themselves. It has changed my life because, in a personal sense, it's allowed me to expose myself. I've always done sessions one on one, in a private, hidden way. Now I need to express myself more. I'm going to teach, and I'll have 20 people here instead of one. Running on the street or track, anybody could be out there. I take that as a model and I'm going to plug it into my professional life. So my mood now, in terms of this exposure, is to teach a class where I'll do psychic work, but with people watching.

Susan: Artist Turns Athlete

Two months before Susan first came to my womens's group in Mill Valley, she had undergone a very traumatic stomach operation. The doctors told her it would be six months before she really felt well. The first night of our class, she entered immediately into the spirit and ran three miles. Susan story is instructive.

Before, I never really felt I could do anything athletic. I call myself an artist-teacher. I make things in clay, teach ceramics, and coordinate classes at the Art Coop, which is an artists' cooperative run by artists and craftspeople. Before I started training, I was doing a lot of functional objects, like place settings. Now I'm doing more nonfunctional objects, like art about myself.

Recently, for a show, I did two masks of my face. I put my face on a color copying machine and then put the color copies of my face on the inside of each mask, picking up the colors with a glazed edge. I called it *Both Sides*. I was really dealing with being a woman. I was using the old idea, "your face is your fortune," and asking, "What's behind the mask?" I realized that my face isn't a mask. I am the same inside as what I present externally to the world.

I also did an actual cast of my breasts. Although it's realistic in front, when you turn it around you see a whole inside world of mountains and trees and beautiful things. That's what I'm dealing with in art, making inner beauty apparent on the outside.

I see now that I can run, I can teach, do my art, and all kinds of things. I'm really feeling wonderful about the feminine principle. I've been involved a little in the women's movement, but I don't like the way some women put down the feminine. I like aesthetic beauty, softness, looking good. I like the idea of looking good without necessarily being seductive. I love beautiful clothes. I hate to see people in that cult of torn dungarees and dirty shirts. There are so many beautiful things people can put on their bodies to make themselves living art. I feel I should present myself to the world as beautiful. I used to see the beautiful thing in my life as art, the things I was creating. Now I just see my whole life as a piece of art, a dance.

Awakening the Goddess

As I write about these women, the flow of the psyches of the hundreds of women I have encountered in my years as a coach blend into a stream of reverence, devotion, and incredible tenderness.

One of the most beautiful side-effects of a woman's training is that, as she plays the edges of her physical power and her inner power, she dares to risk in all other areas of her life. I'm sure that with the relinquishment of the inner fear of her physical vulnerability, there is a concomitant manifestation of her outer strength in dealing with external unknowns. Many of my students have relinquished interpersonal relationships and unsatisfactory jobs and have taken a quantum leap to a new vocation as a result of a Lifestyle Training Program.

Women are now standing up for their own personal rights against overwhelming power networks both in the family and in the business world. Many are becoming assertive, but in a loving, centered way that comes from internal strength and personal integrity. They have reowned their power.

One of the most important purposes of a Lifestyle Training Program for a woman is to help her develop a sense of love for her body, to help her bring along her sexuality and a deeply imbedded sense of being the fertility goddess of the race, with or without children.

Female Transformers

The full spectrum of female energies is reawakening in our culture. We are resurrecting the mythical and archetypal energies, buried deep in our sub-conscious mind, that were squeezed out by social and cultural norms of male domination. As Robert Bly points out, "When the ancient world fell, men took away almost all the women's transformers." As we women venture into the New Age, we have few role models, no path of ego-ideal to follow. We must recreate our sense of self. Part of that resurrection is by identification with the ancient mythical goddesses.

Demeter, the symbol of motherhood, food, fertility, is rooted in earth mysteries. "The Demeter energy transformed the woman's energy to such a high intensity that it broke through the house and was carried out into the universe in the yin-yang way." The Demeter woman was firmly rooted in feeding, in earth mysteries, in nutrition, and at the same instant was out of the house.

Athene is the symbol of higher consciousness and heroic destiny, the over-coming of obstacles and the grappling with political power. This is typified in the woman executive such as Rose Thorne and Peggy Taylor.

Aphrodite is the symbol of eros, love, sensuality, passion, emotion, and supplier of the energy to facilitate psychic and soul growth. Aphrodite is also the symbol of the union of male and female.

Artemis is the symbol of the *wildness in women*, close to the forest, animals, preserving the untamed spirit in women, the heroic quality of self-surviv-al. As a New Age Coach I have subconsciously represented this energy to many women. The resurgence of women in athletics through the spirit of the Artemis transformer also accounts for the rising interest of women in running and sports.

Freeing the Goddess

A Lifestyle Training Program can help a woman free the goddess within, a goddess capable of love and appreciating physical beauty and radiant health. The view of women in beauty magazines is only a facade. The New Age is redefining the meaning. As Terry says, "We women have a sense of our own special mission, but coming from a place of self-will, to better our *consciousness*, become more heroic. Yoga, dance, running, are just the means to sculpt our inner beauty."

The women in this chapter are all becoming goddesses of the New Age. They see beauty as an internal state of being. They are in touch with the universal life flow, doing meaningful work in the world, struggling with self-doubt to create new kinds of love relationships. They are not afraid of expanding, searching, enduring the stress of re-sculpting their *will to meaning*.

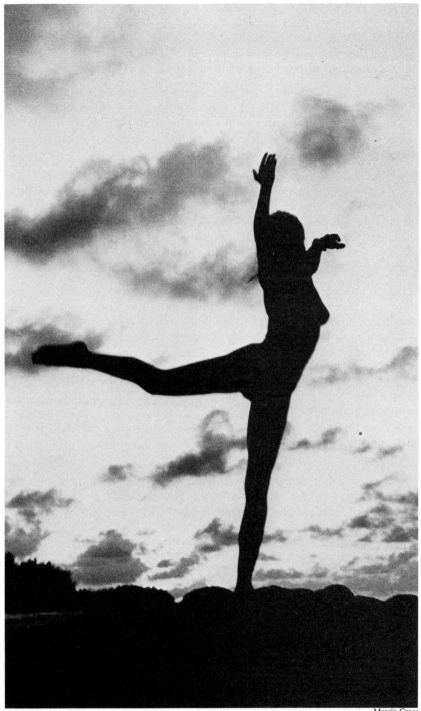

Marcia Cross

All have developed a sense of sisterhood/brotherhood not based on competition or control. They are actively doing their part in keeping their bodies unpolluted, their minds enlightened, and their network of influence aware of their responsibility on this planet. As Peggy says, they have overcome denial and realize that what *they* do makes a difference.

All are now involved in a physical training program with an immense sense of personal and planetary responsibility. They have no records to break. They only have their own inner being to perfect. Each is totally unique. Each has her own style and system. All of these women are goddesses of a New Age *in training*.

Peggy is a heroine in her own personal right as she edits a magazine, making a statement of her will and empowering others to do likewise. Mary and Dottie have been awakening themselves and other women to their inner beauty and power. Carolyn and Donna envision a world transformed through their lives and their children. They see internal joy and self-discipline as their link to a better world. Vinita has extended her personal search for spiritual truth to guide her as an athlete/healer/teacher.

Susan has redefined her artistry to include all the things that the body can do. She is a political organizer in Berkeley, and through her radiance and charm is a New Age goddess. Terry floats as she dances with the spirit of Athene and Aphrodite inside her. Stevanne, with her flair for the dramatic, her intellectually dynamic mind, is a mover, a doer, an inspirer. She is a high priestess with great internal power who dares to be as fragile as a butterfly. Helen Palmer has developed the highest faculties of intuitive wisdom and holds a candle to light the way for the rest of us. Pat Ellsberg, one of the truly heroic women of our age, has survived the trauma that came when her husband, Daniel, dared to speak for the truth. She has gone on to rebuild from her own center a lighted, intelligent career with spiritual integrity.

My personal dream is to see our culture filled with such goddesses: strong, powerful, graceful, sensuous, intelligent, able to retain their flowing receptivity, their intuitive and mystical femininity, while balanced with the skills to master the intricacies of our industrial society. My dream is to see these goddesses running corporations, magazines, holding seats of political power, managing financial institutions, raising loving, aligned children with unpolluted bodies.

My dream is to see thousands of women doing subtle battle and overt battle against the commercial establishment that is profiting from the exploitation of their sexuality, and killing the life force with toxicity, pollutants, and garbage food. My dream is to see a culture of goddesses who love and believe in themselves, who trust their own unique path to beauty; goddesses who feel the flow of civilization through their blood cells. Such women will create a transformed human specie. Such women are destined to be the coaches of a transformed society.

Reowning your power as a woman is essentially awakening the goddess within. This is possible for you. I only hope the search, struggle, vision, and courage of these women can inspire you. Remember, you have many friends all around you to encourage you. You will probably become a New Age Coach in your own unique way. By awakening the goddess in yourself, you will teach the way by your essence.

Chapter Ten:
New Age Graduate
Training

Sports, games, and physical training should help to awaken and increase our desire to reach toward the upper limits of health and fitness. The preceding chapters have provided the information necessary to set up a basic Lifestyle Training Program. But that is only the beginning. Once you start the process of building endurance on an aligned, flexible, strong body, and once you have cleaned up your nutrition and have begun to develop the powers of your mind through innerspace work, you will almost certainly gravitate toward a quest for an even greater transformation of your body and spirit. In this chapter I want introduce you to the fine tuning that you can use to help you play and stay at the upper limits of optimal health. I call this New Age Graduate Training.

Biological Medicine: The Healing Science of Tomorrow

Dr. Paavo Airola graphically describes the need for a different approach to health incorporating *new modalities*

> The healing science of today is in a state of utter chaos. The orthodox, allopathic medicine, misdirected by the fallacious Pasteurian concept of disease and consequently relying on drugs and surgery in its effort to conquer illness, has entered a vicious cycle. The complete fiasco of today's medicine is evidenced by the fact that in spite of more doctors, more hospitals, and more money spent on health than at any time in man's history (more than 60 billion dollars a year!), we have more dis-

eases then ever before. And we are witnessing a catastrophic increase in all the chronic degenerative conditions including heart disease and cancer. Already *one half* of the American people are chronically ill. Our mortality rate is increasing; it is now about 50th among the world's nations. And our life expectancy is going down. We occupy 18th place for men and 11th place for women in life expectancy among industrialized nations.

Because of the medical doctors' inability to reverse the trend, people are losing their faith in them. So-called fringe medicines are blooming as never before. The sick people, not finding relief in drugs, are going to chiropractors, osteopaths, naturopaths, spiritual healers, physiotherapists, herbalists, nutritionists, drugless healers, Christian Science, etc. Or they take their health into their own hands and try to improve it with better nutrition, health foods, food supplements, vitamins and exercise. (*Are You Confused?*, Paavo Airola.)

Self-Monitoring

In this chapter, we will first look at some of the diagnostic tools available to help you to monitor your own personal health needs. Then we will discuss some of the healing modalities available through practitioners.

It is not possible in one chapter to discuss all the many and varied New Age healing therapies and diagnostic tools. I am going to present those with which I am personally familiar and have used in my own life and the lives of my clients. To help you better evaluate their applicability to your life, I will give some examples and references.

Instead of viewing the body as a system that develops pathology and needs specific specialists to diagnose illness and prescribe drugs, the new healing modalities emphasize that the body is a system of energy. The entire functioning of the body/mind/spirit must be considered as either in or out of balance. When it is out of balance, illness develops. When it is in balance, it is healthy.

The Body as System of Energy

Chi Flow or Prana

According to the Chinese tradition, whenever the Chi flow along the meridians is either obstructed or weakened, the likelihood of sickness is increased. (*The Healing Mind*, Dr. Irving Oyle, p. 69).

George Leonard gives a description of Chi flow in *The Ultimate Athlete*:

The body radiates several forms of energy that can be easily measured by the instruments of Western science. Each of us is surrounded by an aura, if you will, of radiant heat; this heat may be perceived several inches from the skin by a sensitive hand, and from much greater distances by thermistor and infrared sensors. We are surrounded by what anthropologist Edward T. Hall terms an "olfactory bubble"; individuals of some cultures, notably the Arabs, feel uncomfortable when talking to someone they can't smell. There is also an electromagnetic field, associated with the pulsing the heart, in and around the body; highly sensitive instruments have measured this field at a distance of several inches. In addition, the body is surrounded by a cloud of ionized sweat that can be measured by electrostatic indicators. We might also bear in mind that we trail a cloud of warmed air, water vapor, carbon dioxide, bacteria, and viruses from our breathing, and that all this material, which has circulated through a most intimate cavity within our bodies, is very rapidly intermingled with that of all the others who share our breathing space.

The premise of all the natural healing modalities is that the body is a *system of energy*. This energy is called Chi. If a human system is to function at a high level, it must have a stable body chemistry. Then, for the soul embarked on a path of evolutionary transformation, a higher state of consciousness or spiritual awakening of our Godlike nature, the Chi must be balanced.

How can you determine whether or not your Chi is out of balance? And how can it be brought into balance if it is out? I will describe some of the tools available. While no practioner uses all of them, it is preferable to contact one who incorporates several into his practice, for example, one who is a nutritionist, homeopathic doctor, and who uses applied kineseology or muscle-testing.

Diagnostic Tools

Hair sample analysis and urine analysis are the diagnostic tools that provide the basis for balancing body chemistry. Iridology is a science whereby the doctor or operator can tell from the markings or signs in the iris of the eye the reflex condition of the various organs of the body. Applied kinesiology is used to determine which organs are weak and which are strong.

Chi flow cannot be balanced unless the body chemistry is stabilized by nutrition, and this often requires vitamin and mineral supplements and enzyme therapy. (See the discussion of Hair Sample Analysis in Chapter Six.)

Iridology

For some of you reading this book, it may be a revelation to know that a medical practice exists called iridology, which is practicied by *reading* the iris of the eye. The iris of the eye, properly analyzed by a practitioner of iridology, can reveal where the overall functioning of the body is weak, strong, toxified, or in need of chemical or nutritional strengthening. Dr.

Bernard Jensen of Hidden Valley Ranch in Escondido, California, describes the science and practice of iridology. He states:

> The iris reveals the body's constitution, its inherent weaknesses, and the general level of health. The iris also reveals the transition that takes place in a person's body according to the way one lives. The iris indicates the reflex condition of the various organs as far as health is concerned, what healing is taking place, the reversal of symptoms. A healing crises is an elimination process and requires a final cleansing of the body. You can not tell specific diseases from the iris of the eye but you can read the overall *constitution* which reveals inclinations of strength or weakness, where located and what stage it is manifested.

An actual examination is conducted by sitting facing an iridologist while he probes the iris carefully with light. On a chart he marks the exact places which represent the various organs, nerves, and energy flows. It takes about half an hour for the examination and, following diagnosis, the iridologist will recommend natural remedies such as herbs, supplements, minerals, homeopathic remedies to bring the body into balance. Disease is caused by *imbalances* and the intent of an iridology examination is to prevent the onset of conditions that break down overall health.

Iridology can tell where inflammation is and in what stage it may be: acute, chronic, subacute, or degenerative. These different stages of inflammation in the body can be determined by the color value shown in certain areas of the iris of the eye. The acute stage is white, the subacute stage is light gray, and the chronic stage is dark gray. If there is a black area in the iris, there has been tissue destroyed in the corresponding organ of the body and degeneration is taking place. Treatments are prescribed in such a manner as to teach a person to *live correctly*, along with remedies to correct imbalances. One of iridology's greatest values is to detect chemical and tissue changes in the body long before a dysfunction would occur that can be given a medical name.

> The real value of iridology is that we have a direct check on the patient. We can tell whether he is improving in health or if his condition is becoming worse. We also have a check on the doctor as to whether the methods of treatment being used are benefiting the patient. Through iridology patients can be warned in time for prevention of diesease. Today there is a challenge that never has existed before for the doctor who uses natural methods.

For those of you interested in pursuing self-study, I recommend the book *The Science and Practice of Iridology* by Dr. Bernard Jensen.

Applied Kinesiology

Applied kinesiology is the study of muscles and how they function in relation to the body structure. It is the basis for a therapy called *Touch for Health*. *Touch for Health* attempts to make people aware of how their bodies work: their muscles, their energies, and their lymphatic system, and how these relate to nutrition and emotions.

Our bodies have three major systems: the electrical, the lymphatic, and the emotional. The *electrical system* provides power to the organs, the skin, and the muscles. Nutritional problems, emotional problems, and physical problems have an effect on this electrical system. The paths of this electrical current are called meridians. Chi flows along the meridians.

The second system, the *lymphatic system*, cleanses the muscles and provides a nutrient flow to them. We are 80% water, and that water is lymph fluid. This lymph fluid is analogous to a garbage disposal, in this case for the muscles. It takes out uric acid, the debris released by the muscles, and carbon dixoide. This waste material is taken to the lymph glands where it is broken down into usable protein for the body. The lymph also produces white corpuscles and fights bacteria in the body. Physical exercise is a must to get the lymph fluids moving. That's why walking is such good exercise. The lymph systems of people who don't move become stagnant. The system gets clogged and not enough nutrients go to the muscles. In addition, toxins are not released. These are the reasons massage is so important for bedridden people

The third system is the *emotional system*. This system has certain emotional center points which are important to the functioning of this system. These are the Bennett Reflex Points, or neurovascular holding points, located on the head. You may have noticed people putting their hand, on their forehead, when trying to think, or when worried. Dr. Bennett discovered that this has a neurologically relaxing effect on the body. It calms you down. Remember how your mother or father would stroke your forehead when you were sick.

Emotional holding is associated with many muscular problems. A common example is an emotional attachment to a past injury. The emotions can turn off energy to a muscle, or can make that muscle tight and inhibit it from working. When this happens, other muscles have to compensate. Stress and noise can cause the muscles around the neck to become tight. For example, noise causes an instant reaction of lifting the shoulders for protection. This accentuates the tightening of the muscles in the neck and causes tension in the back of the neck that can lead to headaches, neckaches and backaches. If your neck is tight, your lower back will tend to get tight, because the two are related.

In applied kinesiology, muscle testing is used to locate inhibitions in the body. By using a muscle resistance test for a specific muscle, you can determine the degree to which the muscle is turned on. If a muscle is not turned on, i.e., weak at some point, you can trace the meridian involved. If this tracing strengthens the muscle, then we know the weakness was a block in the meridian. We have activated the lymph flow of the muscle thereby reactivating it.

By testing various muscles and locating the inhibited ones, a correction can be made, and the muscle will go back into action, thus reducing stress. The problem is not so much the weak muscle as it is the muscles that have to compensate for the weak muscle. The compensating muscles will have a different pull at their point of origin or insertion, and more muscles will go into stress. This causes your structure to degrade, and with it your posture.

Kinesiology is a preventive technique. It is often practiced by chiropractors under a separate license. Kinesiology helps to pinpoint whether a problem is emotional, nutritional, or structural. It is important to find a physician who practices kinesiology since this indicates that he or she is interested in the holistic approach to medicine: the emotions, the structure of the body, and nutrition.

Our thoughts have a lot to do with our energy or *life force*. When a person dies, this *life force* or energy is gone. The Orientals have tapped into energy through acupuncture, Tai Chi, and the martial arts. They have learned to work with energy, Chi, prana.

Methods to Balance Chi

There are several methods of balancing the Chi flow.

Cross-Crawl Exercises

When we are born, the brain and the nerve system are disorganized. Organization and education begin immediately and continue through all the stages of development from the crib to creeping, crawling, walking, and running.

Our controlling nerve system has two halves. The right side of the brain controls the left side of the body and the left side of the brain controls the right side of the body. By the 5th to the 8th year of life, the crossing mechanism and one-sided dominance are developed. As a leg moves forward, the opposite arm moves forward. This crossing action educates and organizes the nerve system.

When normal crossing and dominance are not present, there is confusion in the nerve system and thus improper control of body function. There are many causes of abnormal crossing and dominance. A child may fail to go through the initial crawling stage, or be placed in a walker and never given the opportunity to crawl. Injury, improper freedom to move, the forcing of dominance, an illness, can all contribute to improper development of the nerve system and lead to symptoms such as hyperkinetic behavior, clumsiness, muscle spasms, postural strain, loss of coordination.

There are certain specific exercises that balance and re-educate the nerve function of cross dominance. These are not exercises to strengthen muscles but rather are exercises to educate the nerves. This improved nerve control in turn strengthens muscles. A muscle gets stronger when the pattern is performed correctly and weaker when done incorrectly. By strengthening the nerve system, which in turn strengthens the muscle system, the Chi flow becomes more balanced. By doing the very simple, nonstrenuous exercises that follow, you will feel stronger, more energetic, and more integrated.

Cross-crawl patterning was originally developed by Drs. Doman and Delacato for the treatment of speech and reading problems. Additional development in applied kinesiology and total body function was done by Dr. George J. Goodheart of Detroit, Michigan.

I have been fortunate enough to have an outstanding teacher, Othon Molina, demonstrate and teach the principles of applied kineseology and cross-crawl exercises at my workshops. Before we proceed with morning training, Othon shows the following exercises which can be done in three to five minutes. Immediately, the group wakes up, feels refreshed and vitalized, and ready to proceed with the workout. I recommend you incorporate these exercises into your training program. These are just a sample of a wide variety of cross-crawl exercises.

1. In a standing position, lift your right arm and your left leg, with the left knee bent, as far up as you can. Repeat on the other side. Keep this pattern going for a minute or so, lifting the right arm and left leg simultaneously. Gradually accelerate until you are almost marching in place.

2. Standing, repeat the exercise above but this time swing your leg and arm across your body. Bring your right arm to your left side and simultaneously swing your left leg across your body. Accelerate the tempo and continue for a minute.

3. Lie down, extend your left arm up over your head and your right leg toward your chest with the knee bent. Turn your head to the side of the raised arm and look up towards it. Repeat on the other side. Alternate the movements for one minute.

Sensing Exercises to Awaken the Intuitive

Nowhere in the lore of western sports are methods to awaken the intutive powers mentioned. Yet, these are precisely the gifts that those who excel *stumble upon*.

There are several *Energy Exercises* which can easily be done with partners to heighten your *sensing* abilities. These techniques help you tap into the human biofield and draw upon the powers of the mind to enhance physical training.

Tuning In — You and a partner sit cross-legged, facing each other. Hold out your hands, palms up, and rest them against each other's. Gaze at a

OPPOSITE ARM AND LEG EXERCISES
(10 Times Each)

1. CROSS CRAWL

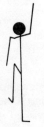 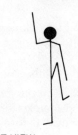 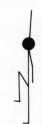

FRONT VIEW   SIDE VIEW

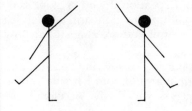

2. SIDE JUMP

4. CROSS-OVER TWIST

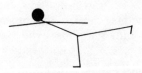

3. ICE SKATING STRETCH

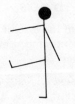

5. THE PRANCE

Figure 16

spot between the eyebrows and slightly above. Allow feelings to pervade your consciousness and relate to each other intuitively. Carry on a conversation, without words. Allow your thoughts, feelings, and impressions to flow uninhibitedly. Convey your empathy and appreciation. Allow yourselves to feel linked together as one life-force. Then visualize a circulation or spiral of energy between the two of you.

This exercise can also be done in a large group. At a "Women in Transition" conference at Asilomar, following a cardiovascular workout, we lay in a circle with our heads together. We were exploring the possibility that when a team "get's hot" it is because they have generated a force-field by mutually energizing each other's Chi flow. The team is moving in harmony with great power because the players are *connected through the biofield or aura* this accounts for the extraordinary power and concentration of the players.

I wanted these women to experience this sensation free of an actual game, and yet provoke the same feeling-sense through the powers of the mind and specific exercises. We formed an inner and outer circle. Each woman had a partner and one began to *stroke* the aura outlining their partner's body. This was repeated with the other partner executing the movements. We then sat in two circles facing each other, holding hands, keeping our inner and outer circle. As we continued to hold hands, we "sensed" the other person and then extended that awareness to the entire circle. With sweeping motions, we filled an imaginery river between the two circles with energy and then stood in the stream with arms outstretched, holding forearms. Swaying and moving, we found the balance point in the group by sensing the waves of energy.

I often use similar techniques in oxygen-debt training on a field with a group of six people. We form a flying-wedge, one in front, two behind, three in the last row. The group runs as a team, constantly changing positions. They tune into the subtle energies of each other while moving, changing directions, executing various speeds and gaits through acceleration and recovery.

Some sensing exercises can be done while rolling on the back holding the knees, centering and balancing in a state of antigravity in unusual positions. To stretch one's powers means to adjust to the unusual; to be open and receptive to the unpremeditated, yet able to make split-second corrections to execute skilled maneuvers. *By placing ourselves in such situations outside the heat of the game, we expand our abilities to sense subtle maneuvers by tuning into the energy field of the Chi flow.* The implications for such intuitive training for sports and athletics are virtually untapped.

Massage

Othon Molina says, "Touch is important in transferring energy from one person to another. It's really basic communication. This is what massage is all about: fully uniting two energies. It's not just giving out your energy to somebody, it's polarizing energy. The basic touch, a friendly pat on the back, does wonders for people. The touch of a mother to a baby is a means of transferring her love and energy to that baby."

As you get into massage, you'll see that there is more than just the touch. There's knowing where the key areas are and how to facilitate, to move, body energy. Get in touch with your reasons for having a massage. The most basic and important reason is that massage moves the blood through the body. Second, you get the lymph flow going which keeps the body clean and healthy. Third, you get an energy transfer from one person to another.

Everyone knows how good it feels to get a shoulder rub. If we can study some of the techniques and find out where the muscular tension spots are, we can accentuate our healing power. Acupressure, Swedish massage, polarity are all basically the same in that they move energy.

The most common form of massage is *Swedish massage* with long and flowing strokes. *Acupressure massage* or *shiatsu massage* are Oriental systems that deal with the meridians. Meridians are paths of electrical current. The meridian points are the gateway to the energy flow in the body. These points can be massaged to open up and release the energy blockages and/or bring energy into areas which have low energy. You can learn to balance the energy through each meridian.

Shiatsu is a combination of two Japanese words which mean finger and pressure. It is a method of massage in which specific points on the body are pressed and rubbed. One of the purposes is to disperse lactic acid and carbon dioxide that accumulate in tissues and cause stiffness and fatigue.

It's pretty easy for you to start developing simple techniques. There are many books on the market that have to do with massage. There are two especially good publications: *Do-In 1* and *Do-In 2* which deal with self-massage. The first is a pamphlet, the second a book. *Do-In 2* describes a system of self-massage and deals with the meridian points, the theory of how organs function, and the energy flow of body functions and why it is important.

Polarity is another system that employs acupuncture points. Its techniques are those that Dr. Stone took from Hindu sources, chiropractic, and osteopathic work. Polarity also places a strong emphasis on nutrition. In other words, it is holistic in its approach.

Natural Balance/Healing Modalities

Biorhythms, acupuncture, and homeopathy are three natural balance/healing modalities that should be considered in New Age Graduate Training.

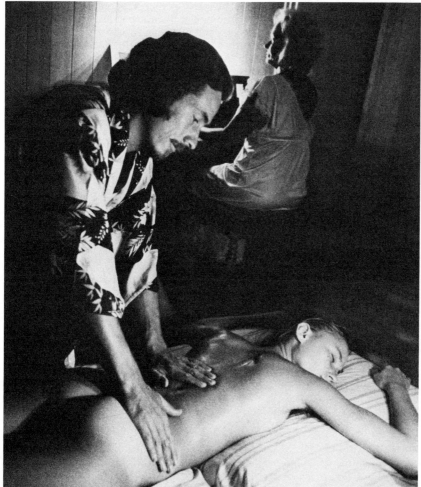

Marcia Cross

Biorhythms

Another tool for Lifestyle Training is the concept of biorhythms. Certain
built-in natural cycles powerfully influence our behavior and can affect our
training. The theory of biorhythms is that a *biological clock* is set into action
for each of us by the massive stimulation of all sensory organs on the day
we are born.

> The basics of biorhythm are easy to understand. In its simplest form, the
> theory states that from birth to death each of us is influenced by three
> internal cycles: the physical, the emotional, and the intellectual. The
> *physical cycle* takes 23 days to complete, and affects a broad range of
> physical factors, including resistance to disease, strength, coordination,
> speed, physiology, other basic body functions and the sensation of

physical well-being. The *emotional cycle* governs creativity, sensitivity, mental health, mood, perceptions of the world and of ourselves, and, to some degree, the sex of children conceived during different phases of the cycle. It takes 28 days to come full circle. Finally, the *intellectual cycle*, which takes place over a 33-day period, regulates memory, alertness, receptivity to knowledge and the logical or analytical functions of the mind. (From *Bio-Rhythm* by Bernard Gittelson, p. 14.)

It only takes a few minutes to compute your biorhythm following the charts and graphs in Gittelson's book. Many competing athletes gauge the potential for peak performances by their biorhythms and there are numerous references as to outstanding feats during *high* cycles. Some of my clients have planned intensive physical and *psychic* training to coincide with a high cycle so as to facilitate breakthroughs in consciousness.

Acupuncture

Acupuncture, meaning needle puncture, is a Chinese system of healing. Specific points on the skin are stimulated by inserting and withdrawing needles. It is based on the idea that health is present when there is a free and balanced energy flow within the body. This energy, Chi, which we discussed above, is made up of two complementary forces: yin, the negative, and yang, the positive. This yin and yang energy force flows along channels called meridians. These meridians join certain specific points. The points on the meridians are the acupuncture points. There are twelve meridians, ten of which correspond to certain organs (lungs, heart, small intestine, bladder, spleen, gall bladder, kidneys and liver), one which relates to sexual drive and respiration, and the other to circulation and blood vessels.

When energy along the meridians is blocked or out of balance, health is impaired. Stimulation of the proper points can correct the imbalances and restore health. In diagnosis, the first step is to determine the meridians which have an excess or deficit of energy, and whether the energy is positive or negative. Once the diagnosis has been made, needles can be inserted at appropriate points to stimulate or disperse energy. It is often used as an anesthesic. It has been used successfully in treating functional disorders such as obesity, headaches, diarrhea. It has been effective in many instances where Western medicine has failed, especially in the relief of pain.

Homeopathy

One of the natural healing modalities increasingly available to maintain and restore the natural balance within the body is *homeopathy*.

Homeopathy is a therapeutic system of medicine developed by Dr. Samuel Hahnemann over 170 years ago in Germany. Since that time it has spread to every country in the world. It is based upon the law of similars (like cures like symptoms). This means that a substance given in large crude dosages will produce specific symptoms, but when this same material has been reduced in size and administered in minute doses, it will stimulate the body's reactive processes to remove these same symptoms. An example is ipecacuanha (ipecac). If taken in large quantities it produces vomiting, but taken in minute doses it cures vomiting. (From pamphlet, *Homeopathy* by Cecil Craig.)

There are over 1000 homeopathic remedies. The homeopathic physican is a graduate of a recognized medical school. The study of homeopathy becomes a graduate program, and in the United States there are few facilities to study this art. There is a shortage, therefore, of practitioners.

A homeopathic doctor must study his patient in great detail. The aim is to know and treat the whole person, not just a single organ. After careful consideration of the background and current symptoms, the doctor is usually able to select the exact remedy for the individual.

Most of the remedies are natural substances made from vegetable, animal, and mineral sources which are broken down into minute quantities to simulate the natural defenses of the body. The patient's own defenses, properly stimulated, are usually sufficient to return a person to health for that particular period of time. New symptoms may emerge and other remedies subsequently be devised. In a combination any single remedy which does not cause a reactive process will be passed off as a minute amount of natural substance in the natural process of elimination. For this reason homeopathic remedies are perfectly safe to take.

This approach is in contrast to allopathic or traditional medicines, which are administered with the intent to destroy a specific disease organism. At the same time these drugs may destroy beneficial bacteria and create side-effects that cause as much harm as the original problem. Drugs can cover up symptoms and in some cases can actually poison the entire system. Drug-induced reactions are becoming so prevalent that the FDA requires that all such drugs carry an insert telling about their possible harmful reactions.

Homeopathic remedies neither cover up nor destroy disease by themselves. They stimulate the body's reaction to throw off the offender. They do not create the side-effects of many regular drugs. Homeopathy's single purpose is attending to the whole human person, and the prescription of a simple remedy to trigger the *vital force* within the body so that it begins its own curative process. It is a medical philosophy which is increasingly being used in sports training in the New Age.

It is important for you to know about homeopathy and to seek out a practitioner in your area. We have a drug-saturated culture and we need to seek natural healing methods that will help our bodies return to their natural state of balance and self-healing without unduly interfering with the *life force*. I made several references to homeopathy in the chapter on nutrition and explained that I eliminated aluminum, copper, lead, and mercury poisoning from my body that had accumulated over the years. Most of us have such toxicity. It is culturally induced by chemical sprays, adulterated, processed and dyed foods, and pollutants in the air, soil, water. We need to learn about the tools to counteract these conditions and begin to incorporate them into our lives.

Another tool for ridding your body of waste products to restore natural balance and vitality is *fasting*, which simultaneously includes homeopathic remedies.

Tools for Body Cleansing/Detoxification

There are various ways to detoxify body chemistry. Just as sludge in pipes keeps water from flowing smoothly, so does sludge in the body inhibit energy flow. We can *de-sludge* our bodies so that the Chi can flow. We can equalize our body chemistry by ridding ourselves of toxins, poisons, waste matter that have accumulated.

Juice Fasting

I was first introduced to the principles of fasting by my friend and training partner, Ian Jackson. He had regularly done one- or two-day water fasts, and surrounded me with the books by Herbert M. Shelton.

Soon after that, I was introduced to Paavo Airola's book, *Are You Confused?*, that literally became my bible for two and a half years. It contains a superb section on juice fasting. I am somewhat ambivalent about fasting, but I can say that it is a remarkable tool to prepare the body for detoxification.

My most successful juice fasts were done in Canada and Santa Barbara. I continued a regular training program every day, and found myself getting stronger day after day. I became more clear and performed some of my most ambitious physical feats while on juice fasts.

I have never tried to run great distances on a juice fast, although many others have described remarkable experiences. I have always lost some weight while fasting; anywhere from ten to 15 pounds. But within two weeks the weight returned. Anyone can do a juice fast at any time and carry on a normal life.

Water Fasting

Water fasting is a healing tool for many kinds of illnesses and injuries. By totally resting the body's processes and eliminating food, your biochemical system can begin to burn out extraneous residue and correct imbalances creating a *dis*-eased condition. To do a water fast, go to a fasting center and participate in a *supervised* fast. By dispersing the accumulated poisons, toxins, and imbalances that have occurred in the body, some athletes have had tremendous breakthroughs in training and overcome injuries. A water fast can be strenuous on the body and *must* be supervised by a medical doctor. I hope the following example illustrates how water fasting can be used for renewal and revitalization.

Following a series of intensive eastern trips which resulted in emotional exhaustion, weight gain, and total frustration at not being able to be an *athlete in training*, I went to Meadowlark, a holistic health clinic in Hemet, California. There I did three long water fasts: ten days, 14 days, and 11 days, under supervision.

Meadowlark, nestled in the desert about an hour-and-a-half drive from San Diego, is one of the country's first natural healing clinics. It was founded twenty years ago by Dr. Evarts Loomis, a surgeon, homeopathic doctor, and something of a spiritual priest-healer. The physical setting is a series of cottagelike buildings in a serene, pastoral setting. There is a small non-denominational chapel, a pool, some therapy rooms, and a series of buildings for artistic, aesthetic, musical, and educational programs.

There is a variety of classes on yoga, physical training and body work. Dr. Loomis, along with his 97-year-old mother, is the leading light of Meadowlark. I first met him when we were both on the faculty of the First International Symposium on Human Functioning in Wichita, Kansas. I was impressed by his radiant spirit and loving compassion.

> On my first visit, I arrived totally exhausted and didn't want to talk to anyone. I was suffering from a depletion of Chi, the universal flow. I was discovering what it meant to be a national public figure and to receive recognition at the expense of my health. At Meadowlark, I learned why I had such water retention problems and difficulty balancing my body chemistry, despite attempts at proper nutrition and detoxification.

> Following my first faster's day hike at 5:00 a.m., with Annie and Bob, I received my faster's kit: ketosticks, nitrate to check vitamin C, a measuring cup to measure my intake of fluids, a thermometer, and a tape to measure my pH factor. I was to take nutri-homo, a multi-vitamin compound, vitamin B6, and potassium.

> Each day those on the fast met from 7:00 to 8:00 a.m. with Dr. Loomis. These meetings had a profound effect in boosting morale. We all shared our journals, recounted dreams, and asked questions. The first day I was terribly weak and had a sleepless night. I accidentally took too much vitamin B6, which affects dream recall. I also itched all night from a ravenous sensation that kept me awake. It was the beginning of the release of toxins. When I did sleep I had crazy dreams, wandering and searching and coming to dead ends. This exhausted me emotionally.

> The second day of the water fast, I was completely wiped out. I spent the entire day avoiding people and sleeping. That night a talk by Dr. Loomis about American Indians lifted my spirits. The rest of the week was one of self-reflection, journal writing, and dream recall. After two or three days, I found that my libido was completely detached from food. I could com-

fortably sit at meals and drink lemon water and herb tea. There was weakness, aching, and some headaches, but no real hunger ever.

By the fourth and fifth days a turnaround came. My energy started flowing and at 5:00 a.m. one day I taught a clinic on running for the Meadowlark staff. My body was floating and light. I had lost eight to ten pounds. I found I wanted to read, contemplate, reflect, walk, and hike. But I didn't feel like running. The evening classes were in a beautiful setting with loving people. I felt I was being cared for by a spiritually dedicated doctor. I had all the stress off my mind. By the end of the ten-day water fast, I had lost 20 pounds and attained greater clarity concerning myself and my work.

As part of New Age Graduate Training, I'm sure we will see a proliferation of natural healing and fasting clinics. It is not necessary to be sick or ill, as fasting is also a means of renewal and revitalization. Some of my clients have fasted at Meadowlark and experienced renewed vigor and inspiration.

Functioning of the Soul

I would be remiss as a New Age Coach if I didn't share the healing modalities increasingly available to aid us on our *spiritual* voyage. For some readers, it is obvious this is where my work as a coach differs markedly from the more traditional mode of coaching. I am often an *ignition switch* to my clients, motivating them to tap the highest reaches of their inner spiritual selves. For several years I have systematically trained my *psychic* gifts and finely tuned my intuitive wisdom so that I may become a more sensitive catalyst.

In my work as a New Age Coach, I regularly consult practitioners highly skilled in the more esoteric disciplines who diagnose the *current condition of the soul.* These include psychics, clairvoyants, mystics, *readers*, spiritual teachers. These people have unusual gifts that enable them to go into altered states of consciousness and tap into information from realities other than the waking reality, consciousness. They usually have a highly developed intuitive and psychic mode of functioning that relates to the right hemisphere of the brain.

I have also participated in many intensive workshops and training sessions at Esalen Institute and elsewhere to train and sharpen these faculties. For instance, at a workshop at the Westerbeke Ranch in Sonoma, California, Dr. John Lilly and Toni Lilly led me through a series of exercises: listening to Brazilian music and performing a ritualistic dance, twirling, holding arms outstretched in reverse directions; tuning into the hollow tones of Tibetan monks chanting in sounds so deep I could scarcely believe they were human voices; then performing a double-hand ritual with Dr. Lilly, symbolically sharing Universal Love.

After hours of such unusual states of being, I was left emotionally over-whelmed, and was catapulted into realms of unimaginable wisdom. The music being played brought uncontrollable sobs connected to the original emotional outburst of the composer. The following day, at dawn, my own emotional upheaval generated similar feelings in my students during a running and meditation session.

Not only have I used the sensory deprivation tank at Dr. John Lilly's home and laboratory at Malibu, but I have trained in Robert Monroe's M5000 se-ries, and have been monitored with electronic equipment in his laboratory in Virginia.

Over the years, many of my clients have pursued similar explorations that link physical well-being with higher consciousness. On several occasions, a student or client and I have participated in experiments to penetrate the *psychic center* for self-revelation. One research scientist restructured his professional career after two encounters with his *soul*: once in a sensory deprivation tank at Dr. Lilly's laboratory, and again following a run on Mt. Tamalpais after a workshop at Big Sur. His obsessive-compulsive person-ality structure was penetrated with such intensity that he could no longer continue his carefully constructed lifestyle. His training schedule became one geared toward self-knowledge rather than miles and times.

These experiences have propelled me to evolve multi-media sensory ex-periences for large audiences, to simulate that which I have experienced in order to ignite the Transpersonal Will and provoke states of ecstasy in which the soul is illumined by Universal Love. I prepared a film and slide presentation which is a direct result of this training.

There are many ways to learn to communicate with your soul: meditation, bio-feedback, programming your dreams, and the many spiritually-orient-ed disciplines such as the Sufis, Yogic orders, and religious groups whose purpose is to awaken a deepened sense of the spiritual nature of humanity.

I believe that these tools are an invaluable diagnostic and revelatory gift to enable us more fully to understand our human condition. Two of the more readily available tools of this type are horoscopes and biorhythms. I have had my astrological chart analyzed and found it useful and informative. Although I have not used horoscopes in my private practice, I encourage my clients to seek such analysis from a reputable source.

Readings are more difficult. One must use discretion. Some of my psychic advisors such as Anne Armstrong, Helen Palmer, and Walden Welch have made clairvoyant predictions concerning my life which have been very ac-curate. At times I have checked out possible ventures and have obtained clues as to how to make decisions. For example, Anne Armstrong predict-ed the nature and organization of my book. Helen Palmer gave a remark-ably accurate reading about my system of relating to others based on my soul or Karmic responsibilities. Walden Welch analyzed and interpreted my horoscope and was quite accurate as to the timing of events, partnerships, love, family difficulties to be aware of. I listen to his tape now and I am astounded. Again, at least one-third of my clients have had sessions with one or more of my psychic advisors and most have had favorable experiences.

I believe that everyone has a potential for these gifts. Tuning up your cardiovascular efficiency, spinal flexibility, nutrition, balancing your Chi flow and body chemistry, and having a life devoted to *high purpose*, will greatly enhance and hasten your progress, toward being in tune with psychic, clairvoyant, and spiritual awareness.

You will be guided and drawn to teachers and healers along the way. Your soul or higher consciousness will steer you with love, wisdom, and clarity. You will *know* who to trust and *sense* what to believe in every encounter.

More and more people are coming to believe that we have lived many lifetimes and that our souls move toward perfection through the lessons we learn in each lifetime. Karma is considered a tool of justice in such evolution. If these things are the case, then readers, healers, and the myriad of such fascinating tools and rituals that individuals and sects use to gain such understanding will be increasingly used. Guides and teachers are all about you.

Do not be indiscriminate or seduced into following anyone. Retain your own unique lifestyle and begin to explore, adopting the attitude aimed at heightening and finely tuning your *transpersonal will*.

Jim Becomes an Ultimate Athlete

The story of Jim Waste is a good example of a person who has gone far beyond the basics. Though he was a seasoned athlete to begin with, the principles illustrated by his story are applicable to beginning athletes as well.

> Jim Waste is an intense, gentle man, about 50 years old, six feet tall, and weighs 160 pounds. He has a passionate interest in rugby. He once said to me, "I could never make it as a great corporation president like my father. But I *can* make a great contribution to humanity by bringing back this beautiful sport of rugby."

> Jim was referred to me by a colleague, Dr. Jerry Jampolsky, who was at the time developing a healing center. Jim said to me, "I'm very busy. I've trained with the greatest coaches in the world. But if Jerry thinks I should see you, I'm willing to try." He was very skeptical and doubtful, knowing nothing about me, the Esalen Sports Center, or the field of holistic health.

> When Jim arrived I had a fire going. I lit some candles, flipped on my tape recorder, and we sat down. He was very stilted and uptight. He wasn't sure what the whole thing was about and probably thought I didn't look much like a sports coach. I told him that in working with people I used some unusual tools, and that these tools could probably help him

as a runner and as a rugby player. Jim began to open up and for almost two hours he talked about his background and family.

He had been seriously injured in rugby, with a separated shoulder and a badly ruptured hamstring. Following these injuries, which prevented him from training, and simultaneously undergoing personal crisis with a career change, the accumulated pressures and emotional problems caused him to seek help at the Menninger Clinic for alcoholism. The same obsessive compulsiveness that he brought to rugby drove him to handling this crisis period by drinking too much. Following his release from Menninger after nine months, he got back into physical training to try to renew his health. He worked for a year and a half but used the same techniques as before. The result was injuries and eventually a seriously misaligned body due to 24 years of rugby.

Jim is married to a lovely woman who stood by him during this period. They have five children. He talked about his difficulty in communicating with his family. I told him that often athletes are out of touch with their feelings, with the finely-tuned senses that can help them listen to their bodies. They are unaware of techniques for quieting the mind. I promised to introduce him to these subtle processes along with my methods of endurance training.

This was the beginning of a series of Thursday night sessions that he called his *private university*. They lasted for two years and, during this time, we worked together at all levels: emotional, physical, spiritual. I not only took him through the basic techniques of flexibility, strength, endurance, and innerspace, but systematically introduced him to the techniques and tools of New Age Graduate Training. Out of this work, we developed a deep friendship.

We began the second session with a light meditation and Jim had his first taste of innerspace work. Then we wove innerspace into his athletic training. We went to a nearby track for physical workouts and back to my house for work on his deep emotional trauma. I ran with him at his pace for a full hour during his training workout, coaching and teaching him the entire time.

During the training sessions that followed, I would place my hand on his shoulder and he would imagine the wind blowing through his body. He totally changed his running style in a few weeks. He began to run with loose shoulders, dangling wrists, shifting the balance of his weight so that he took the pressure off his ankles. He held his head higher, visualizing a bamboo shoot blowing in the wind.

I saw three longterm needs for Jim. First, he needed major structural alignment work. Second, he needed help in expressing his feelings. And third, because he was so bright and analytical, he needed a thorough theoretical base for the work we were doing.

In the third month, I began to bring in flexibility work and designed specific exercises for him. We continued to train on the track and interweave more advanced innerspace work into our sessions. Jim would project energy streamers around the track and put himself in a state of deep relaxation.

Jim began to make significant nutritional changes. He started substituting trail mix (a combination of nuts, raisins, seeds, coconut, carob) and other natural foods for his much-loved sugars and chocolate chip cookies. During this time, he had a Hair Sample Analysis which revealed that he had a very high level of lead poisoning. He started a detoxification process and a balancing of his biochemistry that lasted many months.

I introduced him to Dr. Wai Loy Lee, who gave him acupuncture treatments. He started having shiatsu and polarity massages that released years of stored tension due primarily to the physical abuse he had suffered playing rugby. Jim increasingly got in touch with his feelings and started to experience enormous changes in interpersonal relationships, in his feelings about himself and in his body awareness. I began to feel that it was time for Phase Two.

My first step in Phase Two was to introduce Jim to rolfing and the principles of structural alignment. I also began to talk to him about yoga, prana, the universal life force, and how blocks in our bodies can affect our emotions. I found the finest rolfer in the area.

One Thursday, when Jim came to our weekly session, his eyes looked especially radiant and he was bursting with energy. He described his first mystical experience. It occurred on a run. He described how he had been working in his antique shop and had noticed a light coming through the window casting beautiful, radiant colors about the room. He went out for a run. As he ran through the trees, the light from the sun made circles on the grass and Jim felt that he had touched the mystical space of universal love. It was a little hard for him to talk about it, but I could pick up his feelings.

In the following weeks on the track, I could hardly tell that his hamstring and shoulder had ever been seriously injured. On one particular day, Jim was visualizing light streamers pulling him around the track on which we were training. I was holding the stop watch. We were determined not to be concerned with time. He was going to concentrate only on the beautiful light streamer he was hooked into. Periodically he was to visualize his consciousness moving into the body of a deer gracefully galloping over a meadow.

As I watched him, there was something about the way he moved, something about the tremendous pain and trauma this man had undergone and the tenacity and discipline that he had applied to overcome it. There was something about the wind behind my back, the light on the mountain, the spring grass. I had a tremendous eruption of reverence, compassion, and respect for Jim. I went home that night and composed a piece of music with lilting open fifths and a beautiful melody. When I played it for him later, tears came to his eyes. He titled it "A Thousand Bells." I made a tape of the piece and Jim played it constantly along with a tape of visualizations and imagery I had given him.

Now Jim began to make quantum leaps. We moved very quickly into the esoteric fields. Jim was in the midst of a frustrating series of business problems. He was also having some difficulty with his breathing. I suggested a psychic reading by Helen Palmer. A year ago, this doubting, skeptical, intellectually critical man would have regarded such a suggestion as totally foreign. But now he was open.

So I introduced Jim to Helen Palmer. Helen, the Berkeley psychic we met in Chapter 9, gave him a reading which accurately interpreted his mode of relating to his family and which pointed out that some of his difficulties in life were related to this breathing. She also gave him an insight about one of his business problems. Following this reading, I took Jim into an altered state of consciousness. He sat in a big chair and I used autogenic training to lead him into a cave to confront his fears.

A week later, we continued his trance work. I played Lawrence Halpern's "Spectrum Suite" to open Jim's chakras. I had him visualize his breath as a circular streamer of light going from his abdomen to his lungs to the back of his throat. Then I took him on a voyage to the top of a mountain and had him cast away golden balls of energy. I directed him through various cycles of his life. We finally reached that time when, as a little boy, he became frightened and covered his head with a blanket. It was a powerful experience. Candles glowing, the "Spectrum Suite," the fire. It was total magic.

Later Jim confided to me, "Dyveke, do you know what you do as a coach? You're so in touch with your feelings that you encourage other people to trust their feelings. You play another person's energy system through music. Somehow I've become inspired, and late at night I just go to the piano and let my feelings guide my hands as I play."

Over the succeeding months, we continued to alternate cardiovascular training, flexibility work, self-awareness, and tremendous amounts of work on innerspace and altered states of consciousness. We did past life regressions and exercises to develop his sensing abilities. It was at this point that I started body work on Jim. I reserve this for a few very special people. I would work on Jim's body for two hours, massaging and healing. I introduced him to all the fine tuning of the Chi flow, kinesiology, and Feldenkrais. The Feldenkrais helped him increase his range of motion. He begin to have a shiatsu massage before every race and a polarity massage afterwards.

The full spectrum of everything I am and everything I have learned was drawn upon in this relationship: my full femininity, my total yin and yang, and my power as an athlete. Jim was the coach of his rugby team, the Bay Area Touring Side, considered the best in the country and the equivalent of an Olympic team. He asked me to be a coach-trainer of the team. I started working with some of the players and attended the Rugby Tournament and the Nationals. I helped a number of injured players and counseled others. I would help orchestrate a whole battery of New Age healing tools.

There were three milestones in my relationship with Jim. First, our long sessions of interpersonal relationships effected a marked change in Jim's relationship to his feelings. His lifestyle changed. Second, the body work, the balancing of the Chi flow, the change in his nutrition, helped him to improve his times on the track and helped him to approach his training with joy rather than the compulsive, driving way he used to proceed. Third, his transpersonal will, the desire to be of service to humanity, became much more highly developed. He wanted to put together manuals for school children and business executives. He wanted to make a film about the yin and yang of rugby. In short, he was seeing his training in a broader perspective than his own personal egocentricity.

At the Nationals in 1977, Jim qualified for the U.S. Tour to Europe for the World Masters Championship Track and Field Meet in Gothenberg, Sweden. This is the equivalent of the Olympic Games for athletes over 40.

There are 3600 athletes competing from 45 countries, 350 Americans. Among these people were 2l who won gold medals in the regular Olympics. There were over 150 world records represented. Many athletes were outstanding champions before. The most important statistic is that approximately 35 percent of all the people in the competition started running after the age of 40. Jim placed 4th in the U.S. Nationals for the 400 meters and 5th in the U.S. Nationals for the 800 meters. He thus became a candidate for the U.S. relay team. He went to Sweden to train for the international event. In the semi-finals he placed 11th in the 400 meters and 12th in the 800 meters.

By healing and balancing his mind and body, and connecting to the *feminine principle*, Jim has become the *Ultimate Athlete* that George Leonard envisioned.

Guides Along the Way

I would like to share the work of three people with exceptional gifts who are prototypes of highly evolved individuals and who assist others in *communicating with the soul*. These three have profoundly influenced my life. They are available to the public through their books, publications, workshops, and large events. All conduct small training sessions. I can only give a cursory introduction to the depth of their work that has benefited so many.

My beloved friend Dr. Stanley Krippner has devoted his life to such an endeavor. For ten years, Dr. Krippner directed the Maimonides dream laboratory in Brooklyn, New York, and is the author of *Song of the Siren*, *Dream Telepathy*, and *Realms of Healing*. He is currently professor at the Humanistic Psychology Institute of San Francisco.

Dr. Krippner is a parapsychologist attempting to bring scientific methodology to the study of psychic phenomena. He has evolved specific training programs to assist others in systematically developing and deepening their altered states of consciousness. He uses the full spectrum of education, exercises, sensory bombardment, telepathic communication, and projective techniques to evoke images from the subconscious mind. One such workshop at Big Sur markedly altered the direction of my life. I was able to explore realms of being heretofore untapped. I vowed to give back to Dr. Krippner his great gift to me. Two years later I became his coach and helped him resurrect his health following surgery. He is now an avid runner and we are working together on a joint program for the Association of Humanistic Psychology in exploring our viewpoint of higher consciousness and social change with the legislators of the State of California.

There is no woman I admire more than Dr. Olga Worrell. She is a psychic healer who has been tested in research laboratories more than any other healer. She once moved me to tears with a final prayer following a presentation in a program at which we were both speaking.

It was my first major New York presentation. At dinner, this compassionate, sharp-witted woman, noticing I was massaging a pain in my back, placed her hand in the middle. I experienced an electrical current of such magnitude that for a few minutes I was drawn into another reality: one of emotional explosion, radiance, and infinity. She seemed to be speaking from a *hollow vacuum*, outside herself, as she revealed predictions of my life, work, loves, and spiritual path. She was instrumental in unblocking serious layers of trauma in my psyche by projecting and channeling divine love through me.

Olga performs healing from a distance and has telepathic prayer sessions during the week. She also conducts services in Baltimore, Maryland, that the public may attend. Several of my clients have attended these sessions for spiritual consultation.

Dr. Norman Shealy is a neurosurgeon and professor at the University of Wisconsin Medical School. Dr. Shealy has written three books, *Occult Medicine Can Save Your Life*, *The Pain Game*, and *90 Minutes to Self-Help*. He also directs a Pain and Rehabilitation Clinic and is on the forefront of psychic diagnosis and healing. Another outstanding psychic diagnostician and teacher of meditation, Dr. Robert Leictman, works with Dr. Shealy. Dr. Leictman, a psychiatrist, has diagnosed some of Dr. Shealy's most difficult cases by use of meditation and visualization, and recently conducted a workshop on the subject of developing *psychic healing and tools to communicate with the soul*.

I believe the methods developed by Dr. Leictman are truly on the forefront of medical history. There is no question that sports training in the New Age will increasingly recognize the importance of the *spirit* as needing systematic discipline, just as muscles and ligaments need proper exercising.

As Dr. Leictman says:

> Real healing is when the light of the soul can get through the mind and where the light of love of the mind can get through to the emotions.

> The soul is always pure but it may be incomplete. Therefore, the soul may not be able to help the physical body and we may get sick because of impurities and negative thought patterns in our personality. Thus, any contact with the soul will result in healing. There are three phases: relaxation and concentration, detachment and attunement. The right way to get rid of stress is to increase competence. To begin, meditate on, contact and mingle with the qualities of your higher self. Our goal is to grow; to be better human beings, to live with dignity, love, compassion.

> The real effect of meditation is that it spiritualizes your entire personality and helps you to better cope with life. Some people float around in meditation. Instead of *spiritual sunbathing* we need to discipline the mind to focus and handle the integration between the higher self and the personality. We must tune in to compassion and goodwill (light and love) and direct it to where it is needed. In meditation, we need to focus action, love and compassion to areas of negativity. This redeems, repairs and heals. In meditation we tune in to the most sensitive areas of our own

humanity and train the higher self. Thus, the higher self becomes the real healer. It purifies and adds new love.

Choosing a Practitioner

I always experiment on myself first, and most of the tools I have described in this chapter were discovered by me because I needed them for myself. I usually *sense* by intuition whether a healer is a genuinely centered loving human being capable of inspiring trust and positive energies.

What about the accountability and credibility of such practioners? Some are highly acclaimed medical people with sterling academic backgrounds who have forsaken traditional medical routes. Others have little or no formal education but have studied and apprenticed for years, with excellent teachers and by self-study. Some are quacks, so check them out with caution. Many have gifts they have developed through long years of controlling the powers of the mind and visualization.

I cannot begin to describe the fascinating voyage of personal revelation and the respect I have for the *silent revolution* taking place in the uniquely individual style of these practioners of New Age Healing.

Most are very humble and unassuming. Most have a deep, sincere desire to help others. Most charge very little for their services, seeking nonmaterial rewards of human feeling. Many have effected astounding improvements in health and vitality in the lives of others and have sought no overt praise or acclaim. They do not consider that *they* have healed anyone. They believe they have been a channel of divine love and thus deserve no special credit. There are literally hundreds of such healers. Many, in my opinion, are true artists of the soul.

In choosing practitioners, there are three criteria:

1. Check out your emotional and intuitive responses. Do you *trust* the person?
2. Get a feeling for the personal life of the person. Are they embarked on a lifestyle of health and natural living? Do they practice what they preach?
3. Are there positive results from their treatments and do they perform their work in a style of non-egocentricity?

Summary

Sri Aurobindo describes our goals in this chapter when he writes in *The Future Evolution of Man* and *The Mind of Light*:

> The perfection of the body, as great a perfection as we can bring about by the means at our disposal, must be the ultimate aim of physical crea-

tures. A total perfection is the ultimate aim that we set before us, for our ideal is the Divine Life that we wish to create here, the life of the spirit fulfilled on earth, life accomplishing its own spiritual transformation even here on earth in the conditions of the material universe.

This cannot be unless the body, too undergoes a transformation, unless its action and functioning attain to a supreme capacity and the perfection that is possible to it or that can be made possible.

Aurobindo believes that sports, games, and physical training develop not only the health, strength, and fitness of the body, but also the discipline, morale, and sound, strong character needed for such transformation.

One development of the utmost value is the awakening of the essential and instinctive body consciousness which can see and do what is necessary without any indication from mental thought and which is equivalent in the body to swift insight in the mind and spontaneous and rapid decision in the will.

The Psychic Side of Sports by Michael Murphy and Rhea White provides an excellent description of these processes. It contains extraordinary stories from the *spiritual underground* in sports. Aurobindo has been one of Michael Murphy's teachers.

The purpose of New Age Graduate Training is to ignite you to strive for such beauty, perfection and transformation. Balancing the Chi-flow and learning to communicate with your *soul* will help you learn to live in the New Age of physical health and spiritual awakening.

Prelude to
Training to Live
in the New Age

A person training to live in the New Age is

> *evolving the total self: mind, body and spirit*
> *as an ever-unfolding artistic instrument*

> *flowing in harmonious structural alignment,*
> *inside a biochemical plant of maximum cellular*
> *efficiency,*

> *existing as an open field of energy flow that regulates*
> *self-healing practices*

> *and growing in symbiotic consciousness toward*
> *higher and higher integrated levels of spiritual perfection.*

Chapter Eleven: Training to Live in the New Age

Healing the Whole Person

A quiet social movement towards natural holistic health is now taking place. It is based on the education of the total person, physically, mentally, and spiritually. It is no wonder that this movement is based upon the feminine principle of *wholeness* or *relatedness* and is culminating in the creation of small centers, growing numbers of books and magazines, and expanding media coverage. The movement is best summarized in Donald Ardel's excellent book *High Level Wellness*. Is this movement growing because we are ready to modify and even abandon some of the abuses of ourselves and our earth which our arrogant and self-destructive consumptive attitudes have bred into our bodies and our values? Or is it, as some believe, that we are on the dawn of a *New Age of spiritual awakening*, an age of Aquarian consciousness; one based on viewing the body as a temple of the spirit and realizing our divine source?

A Health and Sports Training Center for the New Age

My dream is to create an *International Center for Health and Sports Training*. It ideally will be near an clean ocean with a minimum of air pollution, noise, and population. It will be a center for the revitalization of the human spirit.

261

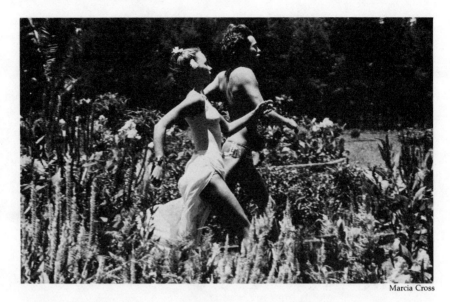

Marcia Cross

Life at the center will be completely focused around developing the upper limits of optimal health and powers of the mind. This includes organic nutrition and opening the senses to aesthetic and artistic values. There will be intense physical training and also literature, great books, philosophy, and master teachers with inspiring messages. The programs at all levels will link the arts with the physical discipline of the body. Poets, dancers, musicians, writers, sculptors, and painters will be in residence, working on creative projects, books, and other activities.

The focus will be on developing the *transpersonal will*. People will be at the center not only to perfect their bodies, minds, and creative energies, but to become actively involved in effecting social change in organizations, companies, and institutions.

Each participant will go through a detoxification process. Each will be put on an individualized program of nutrition based on the latest tools of analysis. There will be an assessment of their structural alignment, and rolfers, chiropractors, and osteopaths will be available to help bring their bodies into alignment.

Each person's cardiovascular system will be assessed. Stress testing equipment will be available along with the traditional tools of medicine to assist overall health and functioning. Each individual will receive a tailored program which fits into his or her lifestyle, sports preferences, and biological needs.

New and innovative tools will be designed and available for developing the powers of the mind. For instance, special rooms for recharging and revitalizing the *Chi* with harmonious colors and sounds. The sensory deprivation tank and Robert Monroe's training tapes, along with specially designed rooms for developing altered states of consciousness, will be available. Mental powers will be developed through visualization, imagery, and meditation. Natural *power spots* in nature will be set aside overlooking the ocean, pools and other inspiring vistas. A chapel in a natural surrounding next to waterfalls, cliffs, and beautiful gardens will lend an atmosphere conducive to nondenominational spiritual growth.

Short- and long-term programs will be available to help people return to health, tune up their vitality, reverse degenerative disease, and learn the ways of natural living. The Center will also assist world class and Olympic athletes and teams in reaching new heights of performance.

I want to help create a center that emulates the spiritual quest of each of us toward perfection and excellence, a center where people will become transcendent athletes.

The center will be a training ground for the Coaches of the Future. As a training laboratory and mini-university, it will have the quality of the ancient wisdom schools, *to teach the way of love*. The center will help awaken the artist in the athlete, to develop the mind as a fine precision instrument, and to inspire people to the universal will.

But you needn't wait for the center in order to get your own training program started. From the material in this book, you can set up your own distinctive Lifestyle Training Program and begin now to use some of the principles that will be taught at the center.

The Coach of the Future

The coach of the future will be a creative artist of the soul, a true *shaman* — one who unhooks the soul from where it is stuck. The coach will operate with the *feminine principle*: receptive, intuitive, "field-force," embodying Jung's concept of eros, relationship-oriented. This will be balanced with the *masculine principle* of sequential and linear principles of mechanistic efficiency: specific stretching exercises, log of training miles, schedules.

The coach of the future must be knowledgeable in the vast array of natural, holistic healing arts available, and realize that most communication comes through "presence." The lifestyle and spirit of such a coach will be an example to emulate. The coach will not hold a stopwatch, or control through authoritarian measures or threats, but will tend, with love, to the growing of a psyche to the next level of *reawakening*. The purpose of competition, seen as an outmoded value of an industrial age, will be transformed: the new goal will be to awaken the spirit to higher and higher levels of personal transformation.

The coach will be the muse, the inspirer of the soul; to awaken the dreamer, the poetic, the heroic, the transpersonal.

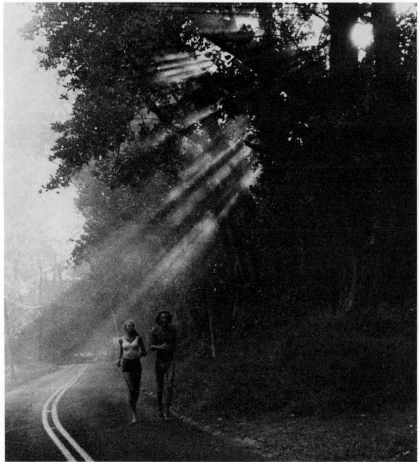

Marcia Cross

Through an inner vulnerability enabling us to be at one with all living things, we can transform our external physical prowess to a mode of grace and beauty. From our aesthetic wonder will come great deeds, not only in times on a track, but in compassion for others and in inspirations of grandeur in tribute to the life force.

The Loving Human Being

The basis of this Aquarian Age is the development of the *loving human being*, who feels the pulse within the blood as the breath of rivers and birds; who feels the air inside the lungs as vapors inside the earth's crust; who resonates with the nerve endings of another's life force, and senses within the cellular system the infinity of the soul.

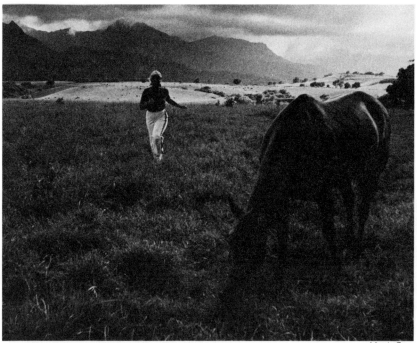

Marcia Cross

I hope this book can open you up to the magnificent possibility of beginning a process to develop your own personal excellence through the inner wisdom that results from training your body.

And nature will guide us with wise simplicity, as once, along the wild coast off Vancouver Island, six sand dollars lying on a log each gave me a message:

1. Become imprinted with the leaf of life.
2. Keep your edges soft and rounded so you can flow with the currents.
3. Remain open so sand and prana can drift in and out of your essence.
4. If you break, know that that is beauty too, for you join your source in harmony.
5. Allow your fragility to propel your powers; for your essence lies in ever-changing form.
6. Realize that in your aloneness you are part of a great chain; ever changing and becoming more of your essential perfection.

Epilogue

As I begin work in Maui, Hawaii on my next book *Magical Moments*, I am also meeting with a group that is forming the Hawaii Center for Health and Fitness. There are indications that it will be located here on the island of Maui. For information, write to:

Dyveke Spino
c/o Hawaii Center for Health and Fitness
P.O. Box 656
Puunene, HA 96784

References

Books

Airola, Paavo. *Are You Confused?*. Health Plus Publishers, PO Box 22001, Phoenix, AZ 85028, 1971.

Andrews, Valerie. *The Psychic Power of Running*. New York: Rawson, Wade, 1978.

Ardell, Donald B., ed. *High-Level Wellness*.

Assagioli, Roberto. *The Act of Will*. New York: Penguin/Esalen Book, 1973.

Aurobindo, Sri. *The Future Evolution of Man*. Quest Books, Theosophical Publishing House, 1974.

Aurobindo, Sri. *The Mind of Light*. New York: E. P. Dutton, 1971.

Cerutty, Percy Wells. *Be Fit or Be Damned*. London: Putnam.

Cerutty, Percy Wells. *Middle Distance Running*. London: Putnam.

Cerutty, Percy Wells. *Sport Is My Life*. London: Pelham Books, 1967.

Christensen, Alice and Rankin, David. *Light of Yoga*. New York: Simon and Schuster, 1974.

Course of Miracles. Foundations for Inner Peace. Colman Graphics, 1975.

Darden, Ellington. *Strength-Training Principles*. Winter Park, FL: Anna Publishing Company, 1977.

Emmerton, Bill. *Run For Your Life*.

Feldenkrais, Moshe. *Awareness Through Movement*. New York: Harper & Row, 1972.

Houston, Jeanne, and Masters, Robert. *Mind Games*. New York: Dell Publishing Co., 1973.

Jackson, Ian. *Yoga and the Athlete*.

Jung, Carl. *Man and His Symbols*. New York: Dell Publishing Co., 1968.

Krippner, Stanley. *Song of the Siren*. New York: Harper & Row, 1977.

Krippner, Stanley and Villoldo, Alberto. *Realms of Healing*. Millbrae, CA: Celestial Arts, 1976.

Kostrubala, Thaddeus. *The Joy of Running*. Philadelphia: J. B. Lippincott Co.

Lappe, Frances M. *Diet for a Small Planet*. New York: Ballentine Books, 1975.

Leonard, George. *The Ultimate Athlete*. New York: Viking Press, 1975.

Leonard Jon N., Hofer, J. L., and Pritiken, N. *Live Longer Now*. New York: Grosset & Dunlop, 1976.

Lilly, John. *Center of the Cyclone*. New York: Bantam Books, 1974.

Lilly, John and Lilly, Antoinette. *The Dyadic Cyclone*. New York: Simon & Schuster, 1976.

Monroe, Robert. *Journeys Out of the Body*. New York: Doubleday/Anchor Press, 1977.

Murphy, Michael and White, Rhea. *The Psychic Side of Sports*. Reading, MA: Addison-Wesley Publishing Company, 1978.

Murphy, Michael. *Golf in the Kingdom*. New York: Viking Press, 1972.

Oyle, Irving. *The Healing Mind*. Millbrae, CA: Celestial Arts, 1974.

Rolf, Ida. *Rolfing: The Integration of Human Structures*. New York: Barnes & Noble Books (Harper & Row), 1978.

Schwartz, Jack. *The Path of Action*. New York: E. P. Dutton, 1977.

Shealy, Norman. *90 Days to Self Help*. New York: Bantam Books, 1977.

Shealy, Norman. *Occult Medicine Can Save Your Life*. New York: The Dial Press, 1975.

Shealy, Norman. *The Pain Game*. Millbrae, CA: Celestial Arts, 1976.

Shelton, Herbert M. *Fasting for Renewal of Life*. Chicago: Natural Hygiene Press, 1974.

Tohei, Koichi. *Akido in Daily Life*. Tokyo: Rikugei Publishing House, 1966.

Watt and Merrill. *Composition of Foods*. P.O. Box 17873, Tucson, Arizona 85731.

Pamphlets and Aids

Sportelli, Louis, D. C. "Introduction to Chiropractic." Dist. by Louis Sportelli, D. C., 175 Delaware Ave., Palmerton, Pa. 18071., 1978.

Nutrition Slide Guide. Dunn & Reidman, Box 241, Pacific Palisades, CA 90272.

Film

"Expanding the Limits of Consciousness." Elda Hartley. Featuring: Dyveke Spino, Paul Solomon, Annette Martin, Jerold Jampolsky.

Courses

"The Gateway Program." Course given at the Institute of Applied Sciences (Robert Monroe). P.O. Box 57, Afton, VA 22900.

Strength Training

Stretch-Ur. Wayne Lee, c/o Hawaii Center for Health and Fitness, P.O. Box 656, Puunene, HI 96784.

Hair Sample Analysis

Dr. Steve Bajon. Dynamic Nutrition Institute, 3340 Kemper, San Diego, CA., Tel.: 714-225-1489.

Training Tapes

The following are training tapes by Dyveke Spino:

1. Meditation for Runners
2. Inspiration and the Power of the Body
3. Training the Powers of the Mind While Swimming
4. Training the Will
5. I *Will* Stop Smoking
6. Tennis Flow
7. Flexibility Exercises and Guided Imagery
8. Stress Control
9. Spiritual and Mystical Dimensions of Sports Training

The tapes are available for $10.00 from:

Training Tapes
Dyveke Spino
c/o Hawaii Center for Health and Fitness
P.O. Box 656
Puunene, HI 96784

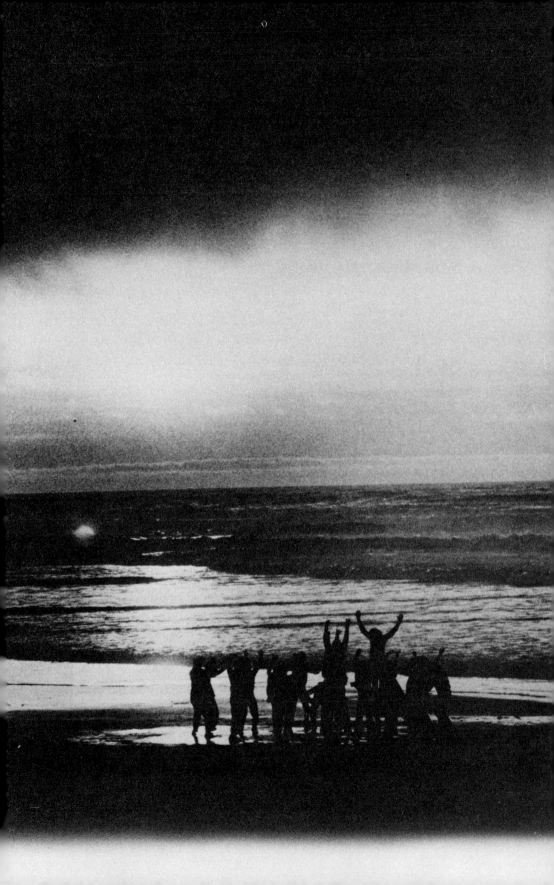

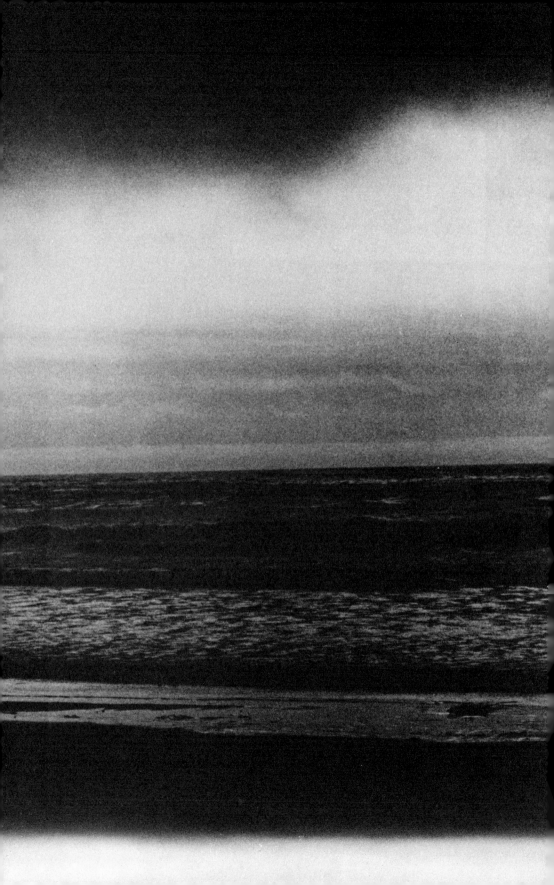